AF248983

THE MAGNET VISION

Magnet organizations will serve as the fount of knowledge and expertise for the delivery of nursing care globally. They will be solidly grounded in core Magnet principles, flexible, and constantly striving for discovery and innovation. They will lead the reformation of health care; the discipline of nursing; and care of the patient, family, and community.

THE COMMISSION ON MAGNET RECOGNITION, 2008

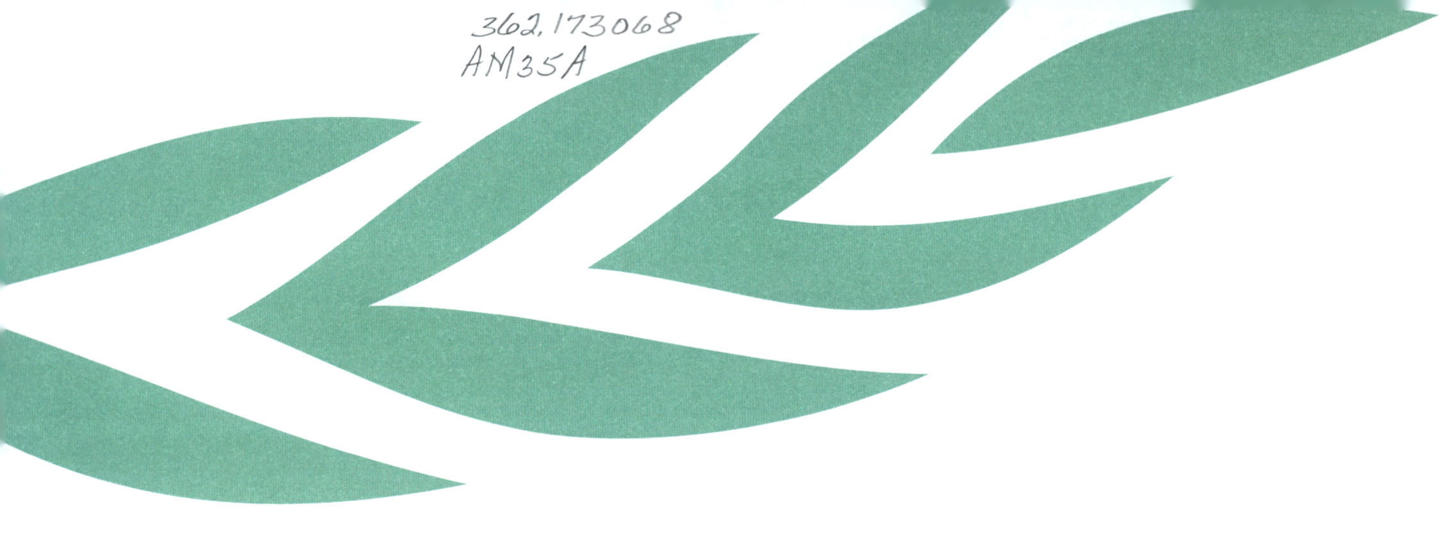

NOTICE

Changes may be made to the Magnet Recognition Program and this Manual without notice. Applicants must confirm that they are using the most current edition of this Manual prior to preparing written documentation for submission to the ANCC Magnet Program Office. See our web site at **http://www.nursecredentialing. org/Magnet/ApplicationProcess.aspx.**

To contact a Magnet Program staff member, see our web site at **http://www.nursecredentialing.org/ FunctionalCategory/ContactUs.aspx** and click on the "Magnet Recognition Program" link.

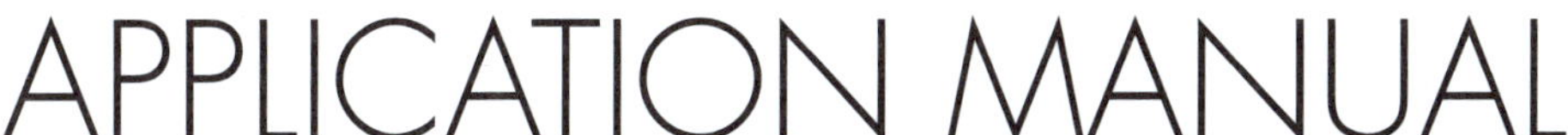

APPLICATION MANUAL
Magnet Recognition Program®

TABLE OF CONTENTS

Preface

Chapter 1. The Magnet Model 1
     Statistical Foundation—The Empirical Model
     The Model for Magnet
     Focus on Outcomes

Chapter 2. Overview of the Magnet Appraisal Process 5
     Assessment of Eligibility for Magnet Recognition
     Magnet Application Completion
     Phases in the Process
     Written Documentation Review Outcomes
     Magnet Commission Report Review and Award Decision
     Appeal
     Interim Monitoring
     Responsibilities of Applicant and Magnet Organizations

Chapter 3. Guidelines for Written Documents 15
     Demographic Information Form
     Organizational Overview Documents
     Source of Evidence Narratives
     Exhibits
     Confidential Information

Chapter 4. Evidence Submission for Initial Applicants 19
     Organizational Overview
     Components and Sources of Evidence

Chapter 5. Evidence Submission for Redesignating Applicants 37
     Organizational Overview for Redesignation
     Components and Sources of Evidence

Chapter 6. Site Visit Preparation and Activities 55
     Scheduling the Site Visit and Public Notice Requirements
     Length of the Site Visit
     Payment of the Site Visit Fee
     Preparation of the Site Visit Agenda
     Preparation for the Site Visit
     Site Visit Activities
     Post-Site Visit Activities

Magnet Dictionary 59
References 67
Appendices 71
     A. Forces of Magnetism 71
     B. Crosswalk from 2005 to 2008 75
     C. Long-Term-Care and Home Care Nursing Sensitive Indicators 87
     D. Application as a System 89
     E. Formatting, Assembly, and Submission of Written Documentation 93
     F. International Application Guidelines 95

Preface

American Nurses Credentialing Center (ANCC) Magnet designation is the highest international recognition for nursing excellence. I am pleased to present the 2008 edition of the *American Nurses Credentialing Center Magnet Recognition Program Manual.* This revised edition is evidence-based and incorporates an exciting new Magnet Model. The Model was developed through a scholarly process of statistical analysis, integration of evidence and expert review. The Commission on Magnet Recognition (COM) worked in collaboration with nurse scholars and leaders from across the United States to develop the new Model and assure a streamlined, outcomes-driven *Manual.* You can read more about the Model's development in Chapter 1, or visit our web site at http://www.nursecredentialing.org/Magnet.aspx for detailed information about the research.

This *Manual* contains instructions for application, writing and submission of written documentation for first-time applicants, as well as separate redesignation information for existing Magnet organizations. In addition, it includes an extended glossary and valuable details about site visit preparation. Because all of our material is periodically updated, it is critical that you also visit our web site on a regular basis to stay informed while on your Magnet journey.

ANCC Magnet designation is recognition for nursing excellence, and identifies healthcare organizations that epitomize outstanding quality and professionalism. Designation can be achieved by a healthcare organization regardless of its size, setting, or location.

On behalf of the COM and ANCC Magnet Recognition Program Office staff, I hope this *Manual* will assist and guide you in your Magnet journey. We are proud of all the Magnet organizations in the United States and around the world, and encourage every healthcare organization to consider taking the "Magnet journey."

Karen Drenkard, PhD, RN, NEA-BC, FAAN
Director, Magnet Recognition Program®
American Nurses Credentialing Center

2008

The Magnet Model

The Forces of Magnetism™ (FOM) that were identified more than 25 years ago have remained remarkably stable—a testament to their enduring value. The Magnet Recognition Program® has developed and evolved over time in response to changes in the healthcare environment.

STATISTICAL FOUNDATION—THE EMPIRICAL MODEL

In 2007, the American Nurses Credentialing Center (ANCC) commissioned a statistical analysis of final appraisal scores for applicants under the 2005 *Magnet Recognition Program Application Manual* (ANCC, 2004). The project goal was to examine the relationships among the FOM by investigating alternative frameworks for structuring the Sources of Evidence and inform development of the new Magnet Model. This newly emerged Model would provide a new perspective on the Sources of Evidence and how they interplay to create a work environment that supports excellence in nursing practice.

Using a combination of factor analysis, cluster analysis, and multidimensional scaling, final Source of Evidence scores were examined to determine how they might be organized based solely on their empirical properties. The results suggested an alternative framework for grouping the Sources of Evidence, collapsing them into fewer domains than the 14 FOMs. The empiric model yielded from this analysis informed the conceptual development of the new Magnet Model.

MAGNET DICTIONARY

domain
A meaningful set of related concepts or indicators.

nurse
Generically, the registered professional nurse.

THE MODEL FOR MAGNET

In 2007, with input from a broad representation of stakeholders, the Commission on Magnet Recognition (COM) developed a Model for Magnet that reflected current research on organizational behavior. This Model guides the transition of Magnet principles to focus healthcare organizations on achieving superior performance as evidenced by outcomes. Evidence-based practice, innovation, evolving technology, and patient partnerships are evident in the Model (see Figure 1).

FIGURE 1. MAGNET MODEL

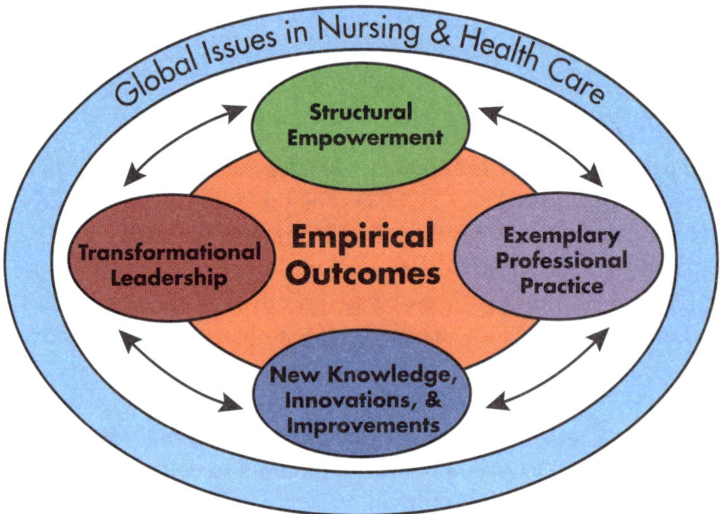

TABLE 1. DERIVATION OF THE MAGNET MODEL

FORCES OF MAGNETISM	EMPIRICAL DOMAINS OF EVIDENCE	MAGNET MODEL COMPONENTS
Quality of Nursing Leadership Management Style	Leadership	Transformational Leadership
Organizational Structure Personnel Policies and Programs Community and the Health-care Organization Image of Nursing Professional Development	Resource Utilization and Development	Structural Empowerment
Professional Models of Care Consultation and Resources Autonomy Nurses as Teachers Interdisciplinary Relations Quality of Care: Ethics, Patient Safety, and Quality Infrastructure Quality Improvement	Professional Practice Model Safe and Ethical Practice Autonomous Practice Quality Processes	Exemplary Professional Practice
Quality of Care: Research and Evidence-Based Practice Quality Improvement	Research	New Knowledge, Innovations, and Improvements
Quality of Care	Outcomes	Empirical Quality Outcomes

The FOM are still valid, but the concepts contained within them can be viewed from the perspective of the five Model components. See Table 1 for the relationships among the FOM, the empiric domains of evidence, and the Magnet Model components. See Appendix A for FOM language and Appendix B for a crosswalk of the 2005 *Magnet Recognition Program Application Manual to this Manual.*

FOCUS ON OUTCOMES

Previous Magnet application *Manuals* emphasized structure and process. Although structure and process create the infrastructure for excellence, the outcomes of that infrastructure are essential to a culture of excellence and innovation.

Simple definitions are set forth to differentiate among structure, process, and outcomes:
- **Structure** is defined as the characteristics of the organization and the healthcare system, including leadership, availability of resources, and professional practice models.
- **Process** is defined as the actions involving the delivery of nursing and healthcare services to patients, including practices that are safe and ethical, autonomous, and evidence based, with efforts focused on quality improvement.

- **Outcomes** are defined as quantitative and qualitative evidence related to the impact of structure and process on the patient, nursing workforce, organization, and consumer. These outcomes are dynamic and measurable and may be reported at an individual unit, department, population, or organizational level.

Examples of empirical quality outcomes are listed below.

Patient Outcomes
- Risk-adjusted mortality index
- Healthcare-acquired infections
- Falls and injuries associated with falls
- Hospital-acquired pressure ulcer occurrence/prevalence
- Patient overall satisfaction
- Patient satisfaction with nursing care
- Patient satisfaction with educational information
- Patient satisfaction with pain management
- Patient perception of safety
- Specialty population-specific outcomes

Nurse Outcomes
- Level of nurse engagement
- Level of nurse satisfaction
- Perception of nurse autonomy
- Turnover and vacancy rates
- Percentage of direct-care registered nurses (RNs) with certification
- Percentage of nurse leaders with certification
- Educational preparation of staff
- Rates and types of staff injuries
- Staff perception of safe culture and work environment
- Staff perception of orientation and/or effectiveness of continuing education programs

Organizational Outcomes
- Efficiency and/or elimination of waste
- Chief nursing officer impact on system-level change

Consumer Outcomes
- Impact of community outreach programs
- Community health and welfare

There are outcome sources, indicated by (EO), throughout the Sources of Evidence, and there are required responses for each outcome source. These are described in chapters 4 (page 34) and 5 (page 52).

See Appendix C for potential sources of nursing-sensitive indicators for long-term-care and home care.

2

Overview of the Magnet Appraisal Process

The American Nurses Credentialing Center (ANCC) uses a multifaceted system of evaluation to assess Magnet excellence. The evaluation includes collecting detailed demographic information from applicant healthcare organizations and reviewing comprehensive documentation assembled to reflect how applicants meet all program requirements at the organizational level. The onsite evaluation considers feedback acquired from public comment of staff and stakeholders in the community. An assortment of site visit activities to verify and expand on the written application materials is conducted. Specially trained, independent appraisers carry out the document review and site visit activities of the evaluation, prepare summary reports of their findings, and submit these reports to the Commission on Magnet Recognition (COM) for final deliberation.

ASSESSMENT OF ELIGIBILITY FOR MAGNET RECOGNITION

Applicants must exist within a healthcare organization. They may provide inpatient, outpatient, or nontraditional nursing services and may be based in the United States or the international community. All phases of the application review will be conducted in the English language.

Healthcare organizations that submit their written documentation to the Magnet Recognition Program on or after October 1, 2009, must comply with and meet the eligibility requirements of this 2008 version of the application *Manual*. The eligibility requirements are listed in Table 2. Healthcare organizations interested in applying as a system should refer to Appendix D.

TABLE 2. ELIGIBILITY CRITERIA

TOPIC	CRITERIA
Nursing Leadership	The applicant organization must designate one individual as the chief nursing officer (CNO), who is ultimately responsible for sustaining the standards of nursing practice throughout the organization. All areas in which the CNO is responsible for nursing practice must be included in the application, regardless of reporting relationships. The CNO must be an active participant on the applicant organization's highest governing, decision-making, and strategic-planning body.
CNO Education	The CNO must have a master's degree at the time of application. The CNO must have either a baccalaureate or master's degree in nursing at the time of application.
Nurse Managers	Effective January 1, 2011, 75% of nurse managers of individual units/wards/clinics must have at least a baccalaureate degree in nursing upon submission of the application. By January 1, 2013, 100% of nurse managers of individual units/wards/ clinics must have at least a baccalaureate degree in nursing upon submission of the application. In the future, the COM will be moving toward a requirement that nurse managers be prepared at the graduate level with either a baccalaureate or graduate degree in nursing at the time of application.
Scope and Standards for Nurse Administrators	Applicant organizations must have the most current version of the American Nurses Association's *Scope and Standards for Nurse Administrators* currently implemented throughout nursing.
Data Collection	Applicants for Magnet designation must collect data reflecting nursing-sensitive outcomes/quality indicators at the unit level, assess changes at least quarterly, and compare benchmark aggregate hospital-level performance of that data against a national benchmark database for at least 2 years prior to submitting written documentation. The Magnet program recognizes that databases at the national benchmark level are not currently available for some healthcare populations. In those instances, the expectation is that the applicant organization will participate in endeavors to develop such databases, establish performance targets, and monitor performance. Where database development is not under way, a pioneering effort on the part of the applicant organization to identify and study value-added indicators for the patient population must be evident.

MAGNET DICTIONARY

beds
Operating beds for the care of patients staying 24 hours or more (category does not include bassinets).

nurse manager
A Registered Nurse with 24 hour/7 day accountability for the overall supervision of all Registered Nurses and other healthcare providers who deliver nursing care in an inpatient or outpatient area. The Nurse Manager is typically responsible for recruitment and retention, performance review, and professional development; involved in the budget formulation process and quality outcomes; and helps to plan for, organize, and lead the delivery of nursing care for a designated patient care area.

MAGNET APPLICATION COMPLETION

The Magnet Recognition Program application is an organization's communication of intent to pursue Magnet recognition. The application is available at http://www.nursecredentialing.org/Magnet/ApplicationProcess/MagnetOnlineApplication.aspx and must be completed online and submitted electronically. The application requests information about the organization such as exact location, type of hospital and beds, various groups of patients served, and areas for which the chief nursing officer (CNO) has responsibility.

Specific information is provided about the CNO and the member of the healthcare organization's leadership team serving as the Magnet program director. Questions from the organization's employees should go through the organization's Magnet program director or CNO to the ANCC Magnet Program Office. The ANCC Magnet Program Office will contact either the healthcare organization's CNO or Magnet program director when additional information is required.

Additional Application Materials

Additional application items sent electronically include those specified on the Magnet web site such as:
- The CNO's curriculum vitae or résumé;
- A current facility organizational chart reflecting the CNO and nursing's relationship with the entire facility; and
- A copy of the tool used to measure nurse satisfaction or engagement.

Submit the application fee to:
American Nurses Credentialing Center
P.O. Box 79120
Baltimore, MD 21279-0120

Completion of the Magnet Recognition Application Process

The final step in the application process occurs when the Magnet Program Office notifies the organization of the Magnet document submission date and the name of the assigned Magnet Program Office analyst. Immediate notification is required should the organization be unable to meet the assigned document submission date.

PHASES IN THE PROCESS

Organizations that achieve Magnet recognition are designated for 4 years. An organization that chooses to reapply may be redesignated as a Magnet organization at the end of each 4-year period. Organizations submit an interim report 2 years after designation to the ANCC Magnet Program Office. Table 3 outlines the major activities of each of the six (6) phases in the Magnet Recognition Program process: the four (4) phases leading to achieving Magnet recognition and the two (2) phases involved in maintaining Magnet recognition. Figure 2 maps the Magnet appraisal process in a flowchart format.

TABLE 3. MAJOR ACTIVITIES BY PHASE OF THE MAGNET APPRAISAL PROCESS

PHASE	ACTIVITIES ACCOMPLISHED
ACHIEVING MAGNET RECOGNITION	

1. Application	By completing and submitting the initial application form, the *applicant*:
	• Certifies eligibility to apply for Magnet recognition;
	• Identifies the applying organization;
	• Names and provides contact information for the internal Magnet program director/primary contact; and
	• Submits copies of the following:
	  > The CNO's curriculum vitae or résumé
	  > A current organizational chart
	  > The unit-based, nationally benchmarked survey tool (questions, not responses) used to measure nurse satisfaction.

2. Written Documentation	To initiate the written documentation phase, the *applicant*: • Submits Organization Overview documents; • Submits written evidence of adherence to Magnet components and Sources of Evidence; and • Submits the Demographic Information Form. A team of Magnet program *appraisers*: • Reviews written documentation; and • Scores the written documentation according to established rules.
3. Site Visit	In preparation for a site visit, the *applicant*: • Posts an invitation for public comment; and • Displays the Magnet application materials in a public place. The Magnet Program *appraiser team*: • Visits units of the organization where nurses work; • Verifies, amplifies, and clarifies the content of the applicant's written documentation; • Conducts site visit activities (interviews, focus groups, observations); • Prepares a final report for the COM that includes a summary of written documentation review and site visit findings.
4. Recognition Decision	The *COM*: • Reviews appraiser reports; • Votes on the presence of the achievement of Magnet excellence; and • Notifies the applicant organization of its determination.
MAINTAINING MAGNET RECOGNITION	
5. Biennial Report	*Magnet organizations*: • Submit a report in Year 2 of recognition.
6. Redesignation	*Magnet organizations*: • Repeat the application, evaluation, and site visit activities according to the redesignation requirements outlined in this *Manual*.

FIGURE 2. FLOWCHART OF MAGNET APPRAISAL PROCESS

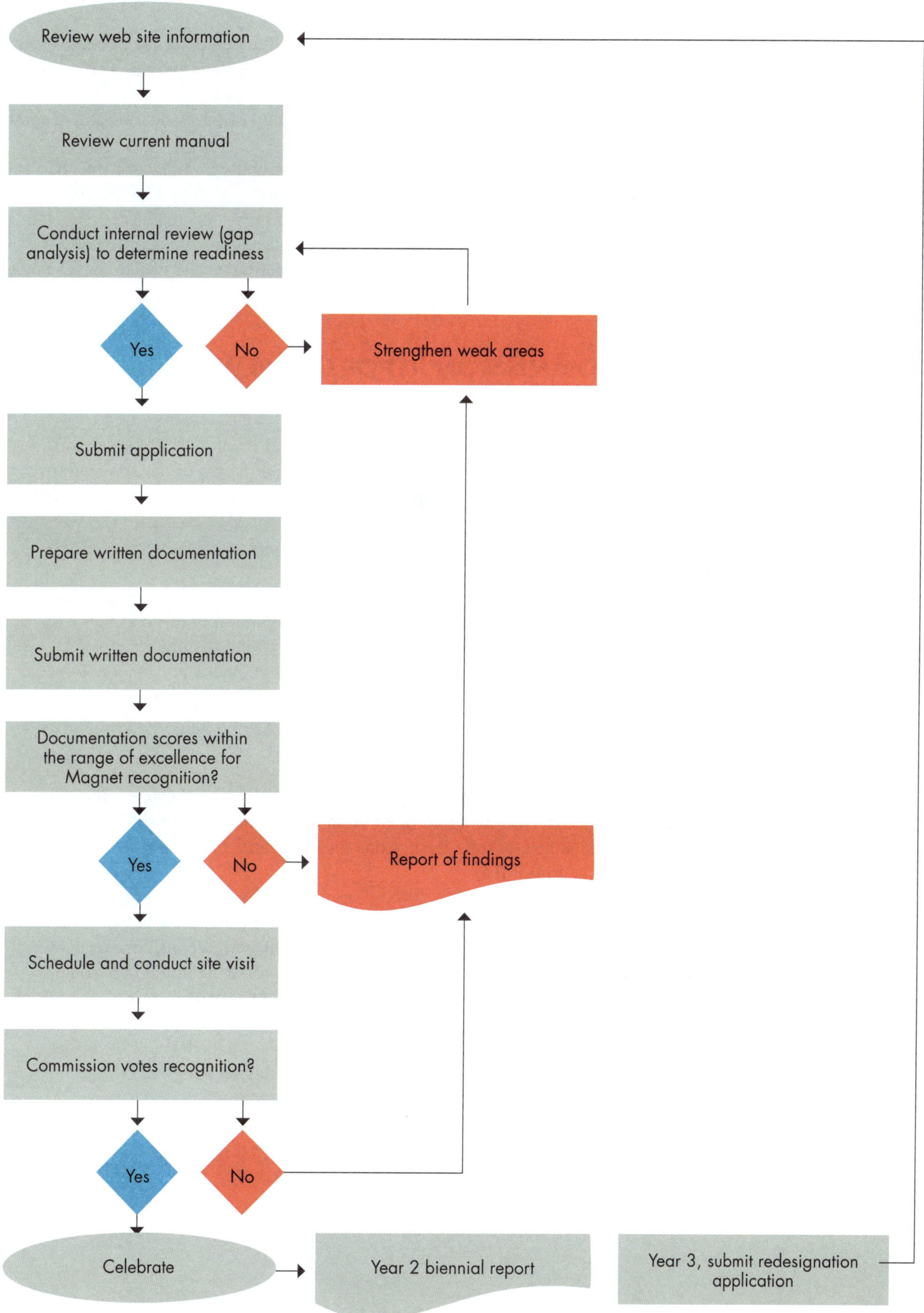

WRITTEN DOCUMENTATION REVIEW OUTCOMES

Following review of written documentation, three possible outcomes may occur:

- **Appraisal review terminated**. Applicants who do not initially provide sufficient evidence to support the Sources of Evidence will not be asked for additional documentation. The applicant receives a final summary of the evaluation and general information about strengths and deficiencies.
- **Additional information requested**. The request is usually minimal and intended only to seek clarification.
- **Site visit scheduled**. The Magnet Program Office contacts the applicant organization, negotiates site visit dates, and provides written confirmation with additional instructions. See Chapter 6 for more detailed information on site visit activities and preparation.

MAGNET COMMISSION REPORT REVIEW AND AWARD DECISION

The COM conducts a thoughtful and thorough review of the final appraiser report. Following this review, the COM votes to determine the outcome of the application. The CNO receives notification of the final COM decision and a copy of the final report.

APPEAL

The COM ensures that applicants seeking Magnet designation or re-designation have the opportunity to appeal an adverse decision. Organizations wishing to appeal an adverse decision must have completed the site visit phase. Applicants may not appeal eligibility requirements, standards upon which credentialing programs are based, the setting of passing scores, or appraisers' conclusions regarding the evaluation of the applicant's written documentation.

The applicant may submit an appeal to an adverse decision after the site visit phase within 10 business days following notification of the adverse decision. The letter of intent to appeal must briefly state the reasons the applicant contests the decision. There is a non-refundable appeal fee.

The appeal panel (consisting of commissioners, appraisers, and the CNO of a Magnet organization with similar characteristics to the appellant) will reconsider every deficiency identified and decide whether to affirm or reverse the initial decision. To achieve Magnet recognition status, the appeal panel must vote to reverse the initial decision of the COM, which requires that deficient Sources of Evidence meet Magnet expectations and that all components fall within a range of excellence. For further information regarding the appeal process, contact the Magnet Program Office.

INTERIM MONITORING

To monitor compliance with Magnet Recognition Program requirements, Magnet organizations must submit a performance report in Year 2 of designation. The report is due at the end of the anniversary month of Magnet designation. The required documents and narratives must be completed and submitted electronically to the Magnet Program Office. If, for any reason, an organization is unable to submit the report within the required timeframe, the organization must contact the Magnet Program Office as soon as possible. If the Magnet Program Office does not receive the required documents by the last day of the organization's Magnet anniversary month and the facility has failed to notify the Magnet Program Office regarding its delay, the COM will determine further action and assess a late fee. The COM's Executive Committee reviews this performance report. If there is evidence of decline in meeting Magnet requirements, the COM may:

- Require additional data be submitted;
- Request an immediate site visit review; and/or
- Require response to all Sources of Evidence when the organization applies for redesignation.

Interim monitoring may occur at any time ANCC becomes aware of issues that may affect ongoing Magnet designation.

The Magnet organization will be notified of any adjustment made as part of the monitoring process. Interim monitoring requirements are posted on the web site at: http://www.nursecredentialing.org/Magnet/ApplicationProcess/ MagnetReconitionProgramDownloadForms.aspx.

RESPONSIBILITIES OF APPLICANT AND MAGNET ORGANIZATIONS

Data Use

Magnet-designated and applicant organizations must give the Magnet Recognition Program and designated research partners permission to use their demographic data for reporting, marketing, and research purposes such as (1) describing anonymously and in the aggregate characteristics of Magnet organizations, (2) identifying benchmarks that Magnet organizations meet to inform programmatic decisions about applicant requirements, and (3) analyzing trends or addressing other ANCC-defined or approved research questions. In selected circumstances, the ANCC may enter into agreements to release anonymous and aggregate Magnet program data to external researchers. Such agreements would be reached only (1) following consideration of the proposed research by an Independent Scientific Review Panel established by the ANCC for the purpose of evaluating external research requests and (2) where Institutional Review Board policies and procedures are enforced by the affiliated institution or institutions of the external researchers to limit disclosure risks and protect applicant organizations' confidentiality.

Compliance with all Federal Laws and Regulations

Magnet organizations and applicant organizations must comply with all federal laws and regulations administered by the Occupational Safety and Health Review Commission (OSHRC), the Equal Employment Opportunity Commission (EEOC), the U.S. Department of Health and Human Services (HHS) or other federal agencies that administer healthcare programs, the U.S. Department of Labor (DOL), and the National Labor Relations Board (NLRB) as they relate to registered nurses in the workplace. The laws and regulations include labor management laws, anti-discrimination laws, and health and safety laws. Conduct by an applicant or designated Magnet organization that results in an adverse decision by the NLRB on an unfair labor practice complaint (adoption or modification of a decision rendered by an administrative law judge); a trial court decision on a complaint of employment discrimination; a decision by OSHA regarding violations of health and safety requirements; or the suspension or exclusion of a hospital from participation in a federal healthcare program, will warrant review by the COM and a determination of relevance to the Magnet appraisal process or designation.

Applicant and Magnet-designated healthcare organizations are required to disclose, within 7 business days after receipt of such a decision, all decisions by an agency or court of law that occur within the year prior to application or at any time after an application is submitted.

Magnet-designated healthcare organizations that fail to report an adverse decision by the NLRB on an unfair labor practice complaint (adoption or modification of a decision rendered by an administrative law judge); a trial court decision on a complaint of employment discrimination; a decision by OSHA regarding violations of health and safety requirements; or the suspension or exclusion of a hospital from participation in a federal healthcare program, may jeopardize their Magnet designation and potentially lose their status as a Magnet organization.

Applicant healthcare organizations that fail to report an adverse decision by the NLRB on an unfair labor practice complaint (adoption or modification of a decision rendered by an administrative law judge); a trial court decision on a complaint of employment discrimination; a decision by OSHA regarding violations of health and safety requirements; or the suspension or exclusion of a hospital from participation in a federal healthcare program, may be prohibited from finishing the evaluation process.

Institutions that have their Magnet designation revoked, or are prevented from continuing the application process due to an adverse decision, are prohibited from reapplying for Magnet designation for a period of 1 year.

Monitoring Compliance with Program Requirements

At the time of application, submission during the phase between application acceptance and written documentation submission, and throughout all phases of the appraisal process or the 4-year monitoring period following receipt of recognition, Magnet applicants and Magnet organizations are expected to notify the Magnet Program Office via e-mail or letter of any significant changes or events that might affect their ability to meet or continue to meet Magnet requirements. To fulfill this responsibility, the COM maintains a policy of biennial monitoring and evaluation of the Magnet facilities to ensure their continued compliance with the Magnet requirements.

Notification of Changes. Applicants and Magnet-designated organizations should notify the Magnet Program Office of:
- Changes that alter the information provided in the current application;
- A decision not to submit written documentation after application;
- Change of CNO, chief executive officer, or Magnet program director;
- Change in ownership, profit or nonprofit status; and/or
- Indication of potential instability (e.g., labor strike, reduction in force).

Notification of Events. Applicants and Magnet-designated organizations should notify the Magnet Program Office of events involving:

- Adverse patient outcomes (e.g., sentinel event);
- Any adverse event that requires an inspection by state or federal agencies;
- Any events that might result in adverse media coverage related to nursing or patient care;
- Any finally and fully adjudicated unfair labor practice charges or adverse decisions related to discrimination or other legal violations involving registered nurses in the workplace; and/or
- Suspension or exclusion from federal or state healthcare programs.

Written notification of such changes and events should be forwarded to the Magnet Program Office within 7 business days of their discovery.

Magnet Organization Mentoring

In the interest of advancing the nursing profession, Magnet organizations are expected to mentor others, which may include activities such as speaking at a Magnet conference, presenting best practices at national conferences or within benchmarking organizations in which the Magnet hospital participates, publishing Magnet-related experiences or research, or contributing content to programs of the Institute for Credentialing Innovation. CNOs and Magnet program directors of Magnet organizations will be subscribed to their respective listserves or forums. Responding to queries from other Magnet organizations on the Magnet Recognition Program–sponsored listserve or message board is entirely optional. There is no expectation that Magnet organizations will provide services of a consultative nature, such as gap analysis or guidance of organization development.

Magnet organizations are expected to respond in a timely manner to additional, occasional requests for information from the Magnet Program Office should the need arise.

MAGNET DICTIONARY

benchmarking
Comparing data from the organization and other sources for the purpose of goal setting and performance measurements. To incorporate best practices into an organization's goal setting and performance measurement, benchmarking must use external as well as internal reference points. The contribution of data to benchmarking processes is an essential element of both research and quality improvement efforts in a variety of industries.

Guidelines for Written Documentation

The three (3) required documents submitted for review contribute information critical to the appraisal process. These documents include:

- Demographic Information Form
- Organizational Overview
- Sources of Evidence

DEMOGRAPHIC INFORMATION FORM

The Demographic Information Form (DIF) is submitted with the written documentation. This form provides an organizational profile that will be maintained as long as the Magnet journey is continued. This data collection should be initiated soon after submission of the application. For some organizations, gathering the information to complete this form may take months because no single office will have all the information required. For small organizations with few nurses, this information can be gathered quickly. The DIF and related instructions are on the Magnet web site at http://www.nursecredentialing.org/Magnet/ApplicationProcess/MagnetReconitionProgramDownloadForms.aspx. It is advisable to download the form and corresponding instructions for planning and drafting purposes.

Consider the following key points when completing the DIF:

- Review and comply with the instruction sheet provided on the Magnet web site with the DIF.
- Use and comply with the definitions/explanations provided in the instructions.
- Submit a separate DIF for each component entity of a system.
- For internal organizational files, document the data sources for each item, as the form will be updated every year. This is important because within an organization, some numbers are not determined in an identical manner. For example, the human resources department and the nursing department may calculate vacancy rate for RN positions differently. Choose the preferred rate, and document the number and why it was chosen.
- Seek assistance to obtain the necessary information from across the organization, including the human resources department, financial services, payroll, and the education and staffing departments.

MAGNET DICTIONARY

vacancy rate
Calculated as 1 minus FTEs/WTEs employed divided by FTEs/WTEs budgeted times 100.

- Consider new methods for obtaining current data, such as a yearly survey of the nursing staff or an electronic database in which nurses can maintain their own professional records.

ORGANIZATIONAL OVERVIEW DOCUMENTS

In addition to completing the DIF, applicants must compile a collection of organizational documents. Organizational Overview (OO) documents may be submitted on CD-ROM or as hard copy. These documents provide information that is essential for the appraisal team to score the Sources of Evidence.

Some of the OO documents provide contextual information and are not associated with specific Sources of Evidence. Where a document is associated with a Source of Evidence, the label for that source appears in parentheses immediately following the document description.

SOURCE OF EVIDENCE NARRATIVES

Applicants will write narrative statement(s) to address the Sources of Evidence. Descriptions of processes or programs must be accompanied by examples to illustrate how each is operationalized. Consider including a combination of patient care and administrative examples. Give sufficient examples from different departments or units that represent a variety of specialties and nursing leadership. Where a specific number of examples are required, this represents the minimum number of examples acceptable.

Although examples are not required for every unit, it is important that the evidence demonstrate enculturation of Magnet requirements in all units and at all levels of the organization where nursing is practiced. Applicants are encouraged to submit data in graphs and tabular formats as appropriate, with qualitative information to support or amplify findings.

The applicant is required to submit a separate narrative for each Source of Evidence item listed. The applicant must clearly identify the Source of Evidence being addressed in each piece of the narrative. Formatting and assembly of written documentation instructions are provided in Appendix E.

Narrative statements should be straightforward and concise and include minimal extraneous information. The goal of the narrative is to explain as clearly as possible how the Sources of Evidence are present and operationalized within the organization, how they illustrate a dynamic and innovative focus on excellence, and how they are integrated and internalized across the environment.

Unless otherwise specified, narrative statements and exhibits should refer to data for the 24-month period prior to the submission of written documentation and to events/ activities that were ongoing during that 24-month period. Evidence older than 24 months may be submitted sparingly for specific purposes such as showing a long-term commitment to monitoring data, documenting trends, highlighting best practice, or illustrating continuation of long-term projects.

There are outcome sources, indicated by (EO), throughout the Sources of Evidence, and there are required responses for each outcome source. These are described in chapters 4 (page 34) and 5 (page 52).

The Magnet Program Office conducted an extensive review of final appraisal reports for written documentation that did not support a site visit. Overwhelmingly, the evidence failed to demonstrate the development, dissemination, and enculturation of the Sources of Evidence (see Figure 3). Any narrative addressing a Source of Evidence must reflect compliance across the breadth and depth of the organization, wherever nursing is practiced.

FIGURE 3. TRI-AXIAL DIAGRAM

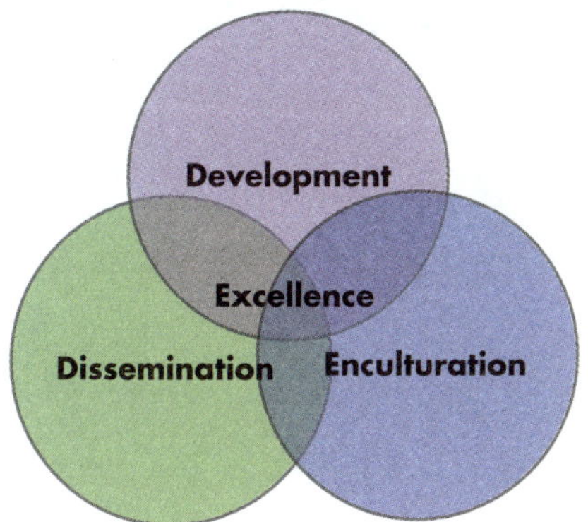

MAGNET DICTIONARY

enculturation
A term synonymous with *socialization*, emphasizing that individuals have to constantly learn and use, both formally and informally, the prescribed patterns of cultural behavior in order to become full members of a culture or subculture. It is distinct from *acculturation*, which is synonymous with *assimilation*, a process by which an outsider/group becomes indistinguishably integrated into the dominant society.

EXHIBITS

In all instances, references to exhibit documents in the narrative statements should articulate what each exhibit signifies or how it demonstrates the presence of the Source of Evidence being addressed. Examples or exhibits must be submitted in support of the narrative statement. Examples or exhibits that are used once must be included in the same volume as the narrative. An exhibit that is referred to multiple times should appear in a separate cross-referenced volume.

Forms submitted as exhibits must be copies of actual completed documents, not blank pages. These forms must remain readable after document duplication.

CONFIDENTIAL INFORMATION

In accordance with Health Insurance Portability and Accountability Act (HIPAA) regulations, inclusion of patient-specific information or employee-specific information as exhibits should be avoided. If confidential information is used in the narrative or as an exhibit, it may be included by removing all identifying information. The original document should then be available for review during the site visit. Where state law prohibits review of a document, it would be exempt from display in the organization.

Evidence Submission for Initial Applicants

ORGANIZATIONAL OVERVIEW

The following documents must be present for the appraisers to score the Sources of Evidence. The Sources of Evidence that correlate with an Organizational Overview item for scoring are indicated in parentheses following the item. See the web site at http://www.nursecredentialing.org/Magnet/ApplicationProcess/MagnetReconitionProgramDownloadForms.aspx for required tables.

Contextual Information

1. A description of the applicant organization in terms of:
   - Mission
   - Vision
   - Values
   - History
   - Geographical location
   - Services provided
   - Number of licensed beds
   - Total RN full-time equivalents
   - Population(s) served

Include an ethnic profile of the nursing staff, client population, and community served.

2. The current chief nursing officer's (CNO) job description and curriculum vitae.

Transformational Leadership

3. Copies of the most recent annual reports and quality and strategic plans for the organization and nursing services. These can be formal documents or less formal methods used to inform the staff of activities related to the strategic plan. (TL1)

4. A budget summary for the most recent fiscal year, actual to budget, for nursing education, conference attendance, and research. (TL2 & EP12)

5. The administrative and nursing organizational chart(s). Describe the CNO's structural and operational relationships to all areas in which nursing is practiced. (TL4)

INITIAL APPLICATION

MAGNET DICTIONARY

accountability
The ethical concept of being answerable or responsible for one's actions. In nursing, personal accountability is the responsibility nurses have to themselves and to patients and public accountability is the responsibility nurses have to their employers and to society in general. "The primary goals of professional accountability in nursing are to maintain high standards of care and to protect the patient from harm. All nurses are accountable for the proper use of their knowledge and skills in the provision of care" (Farquharson, 2004, p. 311-312).

Nurse Practice Act
The basic enabling law in states and territories within the United States for licensure and definition of nursing practice in the jurisdiction of the legislative body establishing the act. It defines who may practice nursing and, to some extent, how nursing will be practiced in the jurisdiction.

care delivery system
A system for the provision of care that delineates the nurses' authority and accountability for clinical decision-making and outcomes. The care delivery system is integrated with the practice model and promotes continuous, consistent, efficient, and accountable nursing care. The care delivery system is adapted to regulatory considerations and describes the context of care, the manner in which care is delivered, skill set required, and expected outcomes of care.

in-service education
Learning experiences provided in the work setting for the purpose of assisting staff members in performing their assigned functions in that particular agency or institution (American Nurses Association, 2000, p. 24).

6. A table of nurse executives, nurse managers, and supervisors and their:
   - Credentials;
   - Earned professional certification(s);
   - Professional organization memberships, activities, and offices held; and
   - Professional development programs and formal academic education attended during the 24 months prior to documentation submission. (TL6)

Structural Empowerment

7. A table that displays direct-care nurses' participation in professional organizations/associations and activities at the local, state, national, and/or international levels. Include office(s) held. (SE2)

8. The policies and procedures that govern/guide professional development programs, such as tuition reimbursement; access to web-based education; and participation in local, regional, national, and international conferences/meetings. (SE3, SE4, & SE5)

9. The assessment for the continuing education needs for nurses at all levels and settings and the related implementation plan. (SE5)

10. A list of the continuing education programs (classroom and/or electronic) and the number of nurses completing each during the past 24 months. Do not include orientation activities or in-service education. Include programs covering each of the following topics: (SE5)
    - Research, including protection of human subjects
    - Evidence-based practice
    - Application of ethical principles
    - *ANA's Bill of Rights for Nurses* (American Nurses Association, 2001a)
    - Professional standards of practice and performance
    - Cultural competence
    - Data and information analysis competencies
    - Quality improvement
    - Leadership
    - Nurse Practice Act (or similar document for international applicants)
    - Patient privacy, security, and confidentiality
    - Regulatory requirements

Exemplary Professional Practice

11. Describe the Professional Practice Model(s) and the Care Delivery System(s) in use in the organization. The *Professional Practice Model* is a schematic description of a theory, phenomenon, or system that depicts how nurses practice, collaborate, communicate, and develop professionally. A *Care Delivery System* delineates nurses' authority and accountability for clinical decision-making and outcomes. If possible, provide a depiction of each model. (EP1, EP1EO, EP2, EP3, EP4, EP5, EP6, EP7, & EP12)

12. Unit-based, nationally benchmarked nurse satisfaction or engagement data for a 2- or 3-year period to include data from the most recent two (2) survey cycles. If available, include the levels of statistical significance as compared to the benchmark. Include a graphic display of the data that clearly identifies benchmarks. (EP3)

13. For U.S. applicants, case mix index information, by unit, service line or product line, for each of the two (2) 1-year periods immediately preceding the submission of written documentation. If this is not feasible, explain why. (EP8)

14. The actual to budgeted direct Nursing Care Hours/Patient Day (HPPD) or hours per workload index by unit for each of the two (2) 1-year periods immediately preceding the submission of written documentation. (EP11)

15. A table of the interdisciplinary committees and task forces at the organizational level, a description of each one's purpose, and guidelines for decision-making. Include nurse membership and role on the committee. Indicate each nurse's work unit(s) and role(s) in the organization. (EP13, EP14, & EP16)

16. Access to the state's Nurse Practice Act. It is sufficient to provide the web address of this document after validating that the most current version of the act is available on the web site. If this is not the case, provide a hard copy of the most current version of the act. (EP19)

17. Performance appraisal tools, if used, and all associated peer evaluation tools for staff nurses and nurse leaders. Include frequency of evaluation. If the organization uses multiple versions of these tools, provide a representative sample for all levels of nurses. (EP20)

18. A description of the process by which the CNO or his or her designeé participates in credentialing, privileging, and evaluating advanced-practice nurses. Include the frequency of re-privileging.

19. The policies and procedures that address patient ethical issues/needs. Describe the leadership of nurses in developing and participating in these programs. (EP23)

20. The policies and procedures that permit and encourage nurses to confidentially express their concerns about their professional practice environment without retribution. (EP28)

21. The policies and procedures that address the identification and management of problems related to incompetent, unsafe, or unprofessional practice or conduct. (EP28)

22. The policies and procedures regarding interdisciplinary conflict. (EP29)

23. Nursing-sensitive indicator data related to patient outcomes for a 2-year period. If available, include the levels of statistical significance as compared to the benchmark. Data at the unit level by measure must be submitted on patient falls, nosocomial pressure ulcer incidence and/or prevalence, along with two (2) (the same data sets as used in response to EP32EO) of the following:
    - Blood stream infections
    - Urinary tract infections
    - Ventilator-associated pneumonia
    - Restraint use
    - Pediatric IV infiltrations
    - Other specialty-specific nationally benchmarked indicators

Include a graphic display of the data that clearly identifies benchmarks. List all external databases used to benchmark your performance. (EP32) Note: By 2012, organizations must provide unit-level data on all applicable indicators listed above.

MAGNET DICTIONARY

advanced-practice nurse (APRN)
A registered nurse who has met advanced educational and clinical practice requirements beyond the 2–4 years of basic nursing education required of all RNs. Under this umbrella are four (4) principal types of APRNs: nurse practitioners, certified nurse midwives, clinical nurse specialists, and certified registered nurse anesthetists.

direct-care nurse
The nurse providing care directly to patients, excluding the nurse manager and nurse executive. (However, in some settings, the nurse manager does spend a portion of her or his work hours providing direct patient care.) Direct-care activities can be reflected as partial full-time equivalents (FTEs).

patient falls
An unplanned descent to the floor, either with or without injury to the patient/resident/client. Calculated by the total number of patient falls times 1,000 divided by total number of patient days.

hours per patient day (HPPD)
Nursing care hours; direct hours of nursing care that are *patient* related, including nursing activities that occur away from the patient (e.g., care coordination, documentation time, treatment planning). This category does *not* include indirect hours, nonproductive time, or all-paid hours (e.g., vacation, sick time, orientation, education leave) and does *not* include committee time if the staff person is replaced by another direct caregiver. HPPD is calculated by the total number of direct RN nursing care hours divided by the patient/resident/client census for the same period.

24. Nursing-sensitive indicator data related to nurse work-related injuries such as needle sticks, musculoskeletal injuries, and exposures (e.g., laser, chemicals, toxins, infectious agents). (EP5, EP15, & EP30)

25. A description of the infrastructure, the organizational committees, and decision-making bodies specifically designed to oversee the quality of patient care. (EP33)

26. Patient satisfaction data at the unit level by measure for a 2-year period, including statistical levels of significance. Include a graphic display of the data that clearly identifies benchmarks. (EP35)

New Knowledge, Innovations, and Improvements

27. The institution's policies, procedures (including Institutional Review Board), and processes that protect the rights of participants in research. (NK2)

28. The credentials or related experience of all external experts and other resources used to develop and/or improve the infrastructures, capacities, and processes for evidence-based practice and research. (NK4 & NK4EO)

COMPONENTS AND SOURCES OF EVIDENCE

This section describes the expectations for each of the five (5) model components and lists the Magnet program requirements as Sources of Evidence. Table 4 depicts the labeling convention used to refer to the Sources of Evidence by Magnet Model component (e.g., TL4 or TL4EO). The Sources of Evidence are further subcategorized for easy understanding (e.g., *Strategic Planning*, *Advocacy and Influence*, and *Visibility and Accessibility*).

TABLE 4. REFERENCE LABELS OF THE SOURCES OF EVIDENCE

LABEL	MODEL COMPONENT	SOURCE NUMBER	OUTCOME IDENTIFIER
TL	Transformational Leadership	TL1, TL2, etc.	TL3EO, etc
SE	Structural Empowerment	SE1, SE2, etc.	SE2EO, etc.
EP	Exemplary Professional Practice	EP1, EP2, etc.	EP1EO, etc.
NK	New Knowledge, Innovations, and Improvements	NK1, NK2, etc.	NK4EO, etc.
EO	Empirical Outcomes		

Note that the Empirical Outcome (EO) sources are embedded as part of the other four (4) Model components. Writing guidelines for empirical outcomes are described in chapters 4 (page 34) and 5 (page 52).

For new applicants, Transformational Leadership, Structural Empowerment, and Exemplary Professional Practice will bear heavier weight (highlighted in gold) than New Knowledge, Innovations, and Improvements and Empirical Outcomes. For redesignating organizations, New Knowledge, Innovations, and Improvements and Empirical Outcomes will be more heavily weighted than Transformational Leadership, Structural Empowerment, and Exemplary Professional Practice (see Table 5).

TABLE 5. WEIGHT OF THE COMPONENTS OF THE MAGNET MODEL

NEW APPLICANTS	REDESIGNATING MAGNETS
Transformational Leadership	Transformational Leadership
Structural Empowerment	Structural Empowerment
Exemplary Professional Practice	Exemplary Professional Practice
New Knowledge, Innovations, and Improvements	New Knowledge, Innovations, and Improvements
Empirical Outcomes	Empirical Outcomes

Key: Gold highlights represent more heavily-weighted components

COMPONENTS AND SOURCES OF EVIDENCE

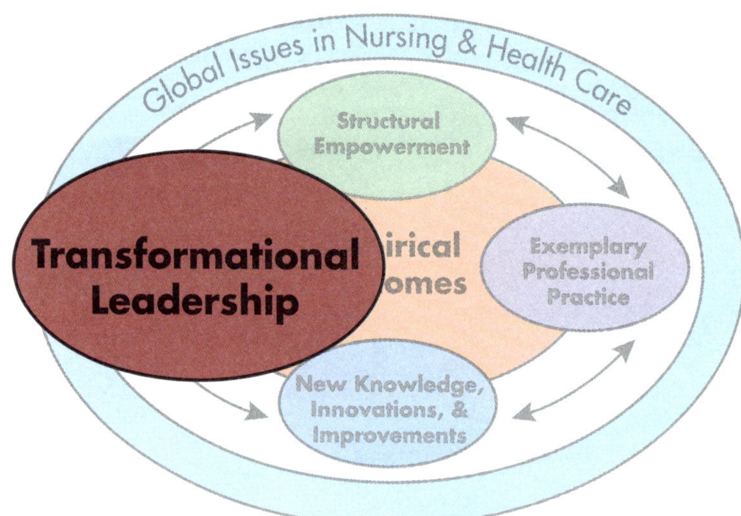

FORCES OF MAGNETIS
- QUALITY OF NURSING LEADERSHIP
- MANAGEMENT STYLE

I. Transformational Leadership (TL)

The CNO in a Magnet organization is a knowledgeable, transformational leader who develops a strong vision and well-articulated philosophy, Professional Practice Model, and strategic and quality plans in leading nursing services. The transformational CNO communicates expectations, develops leaders, and evolves the organization to meet current and anticipated needs and strategic priorities. Nursing leaders at all levels of the organization convey a strong sense of advocacy and support on behalf of staff and patients.

The CNO must be strategically positioned within the organization to effectively influence other executive stakeholders, including the board of directors/trustees. Strategic positioning is imperative to achieving the level of influence required to lead others both operationally and during periods of change management due to internal or external factors. Executive-level nursing leaders serve at the executive level of the organization, with the CNO typically reporting to the chief executive officer.

The nursing organization must be continually assessed, and appropriate strategic and quality plans for nursing and patient care developed that are congruent with those of the organization. The CNO must secure adequate resources to implement these plans and engage in interdisciplinary efforts to accomplish this work.

Wherever nursing is practiced, the CNO must develop structures, processes, and expectations for staff nurse input and involvement throughout the organization. Mechanisms must be implemented for evidence-based practice to evolve and for innovation to flourish. The CNO should be seen as an executive leader and a nursing advocate and perceived as leading nursing practice and patient care. The CNO is visible, accessible, and communicates effectively in an environment of mutual respect. As a result, nurses throughout the organization should perceive that their voices are heard, their input valued, and their practice supported.

Sources of Evidence

Strategic Planning. Describe and demonstrate

TL1   How nursing's mission, vision, values, and strategic and quality plans reflect the organization's current and anticipated strategic priorities.

TL2   How nurses at every level—CNO, nurse administrators, and direct-care nurses—advocate for resources, including fiscal and technology resources, to support unit/division goals.

TL3   The strategic planning structure(s) and process(es) used by nursing to improve the healthcare system's:
- Effectiveness and
- Efficiency.

TL3EO   The outcome(s) that resulted from the planning described in TL3.

Advocacy and Influence. Describe and demonstrate

TL4   The process(es) that enable the CNO to influence organization-wide changes.

TL4EO   One (1) CNO-influenced organization-wide change.

TL5   How nurse leaders guide the transition during periods of planned or unplanned change.

TL6   How the organization supports:
- Leadership development
- Performance management
- Mentoring activities
- Succession planning for nurse leaders

TL7   How nurse leaders value, encourage, recognize/reward, and implement innovation.

Visibility, Accessibility, and Communication. Describe and demonstrate

TL8   The various methods by which the CNO is visible and accesses direct-care nurses.

TL9   The various methods by which direct-care nurses access nurse leaders.

TL10   How nurse leaders use input from direct-care nurses to improve the work environment and patient care.

TL10EO   Changes in the work environment and patient care based on input from the direct-care nurses.

MAGNET DICTIONARY

nurse administrator
A registered nurse whose primary responsibility is the management of healthcare services delivery and who represents nursing. For the purposes of this document, the two levels of nurse administrators are those of the *nurse executive* and the *nurse manager* (see entries in the Magnet Dictionary on page 62).

nurses at every level
This phrase is used when it is important that direct-care nurses and nurses in every role, not solely nurse managers and nurse administrators, participate in decision-making bodies.

INITIAL APPLICATION

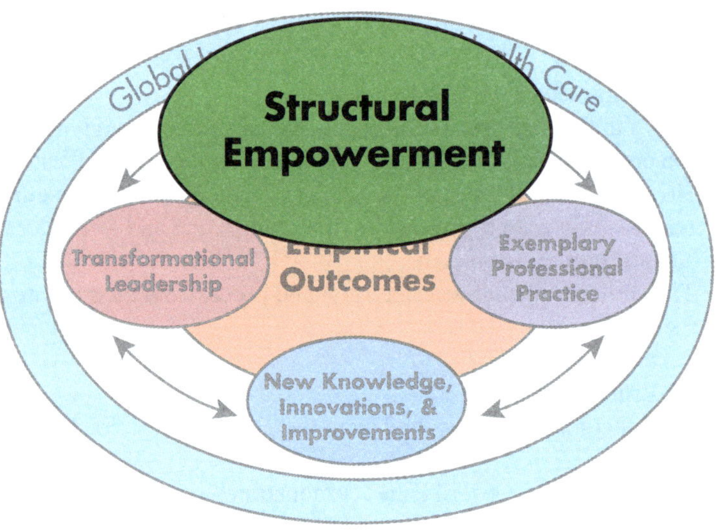

FORCES OF MAGNETISM
- ORGANIZATIONAL STRUCTURE
- PERSONNEL POLICIES AND PROGRAMS
- COMMUNITY AND THE HEALTHCARE ORGANIZATION
- IMAGE OF NURSING
- PROFESSIONAL DEVELOPMENT

MAGNET DICTIONARY

standard
A norm that expresses an agreed-upon level of performance that has been developed to characterize, measure, and provide guidance for achieving excellence in practice.

setting
A stand-alone practice venue within an entity. The term can be used interchangeably with *facility* where appropriate or necessary.

II. Structural Empowerment (SE)

Magnet structural environments are generally flat, flexible, and decentralized. Nurses throughout the organization are involved in self-governance and decision-making structures and processes that establish standards of practice and address issues of concern. The flow of information and decision-making is bi-directional and horizontal between and among professional nurses at the bedside, the leadership team, and the CNO. The CNO serves on the highest-level councils and/or committees. Nurse leaders throughout the organization also serve on committees and task forces that address excellence in patient care and the safe, efficient, and effective operation of the organization.

The healthcare organization promotes relationships among all types of community organizations to develop strong partnerships to improve patient outcomes and the health of the communities they serve. Magnet nurses extend their influence to professional and community groups, advancing the nursing profession and supporting organizational goals and personal and professional growth and development.

The organization uses multiple strategies to establish structures, systematic and equitable processes, and expectations that support lifelong professional learning, role development, and career advancement. Relationships are established throughout the organization and with the community to encourage educational advancement.

Nurse contributions to the organization and community are recognized for their positive effect on patients and families. Nurses are acknowledged in various and substantive ways for these accomplishments, enhancing the image of nursing in the community.

Sources of Evidence

Professional Engagement. Describe and demonstrate

SE1   The structure(s) and process(es) that enable nurses from all settings and roles to actively participate in organizational decision-making groups such as committees, councils, and task forces.

SE1EO   Two (2) improvements in different practice settings because of nurse involvement in organizational decision-making groups such as committees, councils, and task forces.

SE2   The structure(s) and process(es) that enable nurses at all levels to participate in professional nursing organizations at the local, state, and national levels. Include international participation, if any.

SE2EO   Two (2) improvements in different practice settings that occurred because of nurse involvement in a professional nursing organization(s).

Commitment to Professional Development. Describe and demonstrate

SE3   How the organization sets expectations and supports nurses at all levels who seek additional formal nursing education (e.g., baccalaureate, master's, doctoral degrees).

SE3EO   That the organization has met goals for improvement in formal education. Graphically summarize at least 2 years of data to display changes over time.

SE4   How the organization sets goals and supports professional development and professional certification, such as tuition/registration reimbursement and participation in external local, regional, national, and international conferences or meetings.

SE4EO   That the organization has met goals for improvement in professional certification. Graphically summarize at least 2 years of data to display changes over time. Include participation of nurses in all specialties.

SE5   The structure(s) and process(es) used by nursing to develop and provide continuing education programs for nurses at all levels and settings. Include how the organization provides onsite internal electronic and classroom methods. Do not include orientation.

SE5EO   The effectiveness of two (2) educational programs provided in SE5.

SE6   How the organization provides career development opportunities for non-nurse employees and members of the community interested in becoming a nurse.

Teaching and Role Development. Describe and demonstrate

SE7   The structure(s) and process(es) used by the organization to promote the teaching role of nurses. Include examples related to patients and staff members.

SE8   How nursing facilitates the effective transition of new graduate nurses into the work environment.

SE9   How nurses support community educational activities.

SE10   How nurses support academic practicum experiences and serve as preceptors, instructors, adjunct faculty, or faculty.

Commitment to Community Involvement. Describe and demonstrate

SE11   The structure(s) and process(es) used to identify and allocate resources for affiliations with schools of nursing, consortiums, or community outreach programs.

SE11EO The result(s) of the affiliations with schools of nursing, consortiums, or community outreach programs described in SE11.

SE12   How the organization supports and recognizes the participation of nurses at all levels in service to the community.

SE13   How the organization or nursing addresses the healthcare needs of the community by establishing partnerships.

Recognition of Nursing. Describe and demonstrate

SE14   The structure(s) and process(es) the organization uses to recognize and make visible the contributions of nurses.

SE15   That the nursing community and the community at large (e.g., local, state, national, international) recognize the value of nursing in the organization.

MAGNET DICTIONARY

professional organization
Professional bodies, which may be known as *organizations*, *associations*, or *societies*, that usually have the purpose of advancing a profession and protecting the public interest. Many professional organizations include voluntary certification processes among their functions as a vehicle to verify that members meet certain prespecified standards.

continuing education
Systematic professional learning experiences designed to augment the knowledge, skills, and attitudes of nurses' contributions to quality health care and their pursuit of professional career goals.

new graduate
A nurse in first employment following completion of registered nurse education in the United States.

INITIAL APPLICATION

FORCES OF MAGNETISM
- PROFESSIONAL MODELS OF CARE
- CONSULTATION AND RESOURCES
- AUTONOMY
- NURSES AS TEACHERS
- INTERDISCIPLINARY RELATIONSHIPS
- QUALITY OF CARE: ETHICS, PATIENT SAFETY AND QUALITY INFRASTRUCTURE
- QUALITY IMPROVEMENT

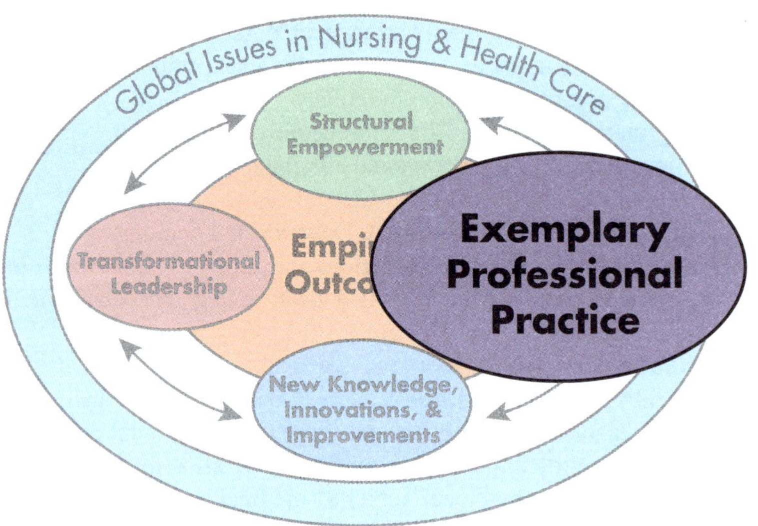

III. Exemplary Professional Practice (EP)

A Professional Practice Model is the overarching conceptual framework for nurses, nursing care, and interdisciplinary patient care. It is a schematic description of a system, theory, or phenomenon that depicts how nurses practice, collaborate, communicate, and develop professionally to provide the highest quality care for those served by the organization (e.g., patients, families, community). The Professional Practice Model illustrates the alignment and integration of nursing practice with the mission, vision, philosophy, and values that nursing has adapted. Magnet hospitals take the lead in research efforts to create and test models of professional practice for nurses.

The Care Delivery System is integrated within the Professional Practice Model and promotes continuous, consistent, efficient, and accountable delivery of nursing care. The Care Delivery System is adapted to regulatory considerations and describes the manner in which care is delivered, skill set required, context of care, and expected outcomes of care. Nurses create patient care delivery systems that delineate the nurses' authority and accountability for clinical decision-making and outcomes. At the organizational level, nurse leaders ensure that care is patient/family centered.

Exemplary professional practice is evident in Magnet hospitals. Nurses have significant control over staffing and scheduling processes and work in collaboration with interdisciplinary partners to achieve high-quality patient outcomes.

Interdisciplinary collaboration is evident with clear expectations and direction to all practicing nurses about the importance of partnerships with patients and families, and with the disciplines of medicine, pharmacy, nutrition, rehabilitation, social work, psychology, and other professions to ensure a comprehensive care plan. Collegial working relationships within and among the disciplines are valued by the organization and its employees. Mutual respect is based on the premise that all members of the healthcare team make essential and meaningful contributions in the achievement of clinical outcomes. Conflict management strategies are in place and used effectively, when indicated.

The autonomous nurse makes judgments about how to provide care based on the unique needs and attributes of the patient and family. The knowledge, skills, and resources that have been identified by the nursing staff as necessary to practice are consistently available in the practice environment. These resources form the basis of the Care Delivery System. Competency assessment and peer evaluation ensures that the nurse bases care delivery decisions on current evidence about safe and ethical practice using the nursing process.

Attention is given to achieving equity in care. Workplace advocacy initiatives address ethical issues and the privacy, security, and confidentiality of patients and staff.

The achievement of exemplary professional practice is grounded by a culture of safety, quality monitoring, and quality improvement. Nurses collaborate with other disciplines to ensure that care is comprehensive, coordinated, and monitored for effectiveness through the quality improvement model. Nurses participate in safety initiatives that incorporate national best practices. Sufficient resources are available to respond to safety initiatives and quality improvements for patients and employees.

Nurses at all levels analyze data and use national benchmarks to gain a comparative perspective about their performance and the care patients receive. Action plans are developed that lead to systematic improvements over time. Magnet hospital data demonstrate outcome measures that outperform the benchmark statistic of the national database used in patient and nursing-sensitive indicators the majority of the time.

Sources of Evidence

Professional Practice Model. Describe and demonstrate

EP1	How nurses develop, apply, evaluate, adapt, and modify the Professional Practice Model.
EP1EO	The result(s) of applying the Professional Practice Model. Include two (2) examples related to nursing practice, collaboration, communication, or professional development activities.
EP2	How nurses investigate, develop, implement, and systematically evaluate standards of practice and standards of care.
EP3	The structure(s) and process(es) that include direct-care nurse involvement in tracking and analyzing nurse satisfaction or engagement data.
EP3EO	That nurse satisfaction or engagement data aggregated at the organization or unit level outperform the mean, median or other benchmark statistic of the national database used. Include participation rates, analysis, and evaluation of the data.

Care Delivery System(s). Describe and demonstrate

EP4	That the structure(s) and process(es) of the Care Delivery System(s) involve the patient and/or his or her support system in the planning and delivery of care. Provide at least two (2) examples of a plan of care that included patient and/or family member involvement.
EP5	How nurses use the Care Delivery System(s) to make patient care assignments that ensure continuity, quality, and effectiveness of care within and across services and settings.
EP6	How regulatory and professional standards are incorporated into the Care Delivery System(s).
EP7	The structure(s) and process(es) used to engage internal experts and external consultants to improve care in the practice setting.
EP7EO	Two (2) improvements in the practice setting that occurred as a result of the use of internal experts or external consultants.

Staffing, Scheduling, and Budgeting Processes. Describe and demonstrate

EP8 How nurses use trended data to formulate the staffing plan and acquire necessary resources to assure consistent application of the Care Delivery System(s).

EP9 How direct-care nurses participate in staffing and scheduling processes.

EP10 How nurses develop, implement, and evaluate action plans related to unit-based staff recruitment and retention.

EP11 How guidelines such as the *ANA Principles of Nurse Staffing* (American Nurses Association, 2005), standards for scheduling, delegation, and from nursing specialty organizations and/or state-mandated requirements are incorporated into staffing and scheduling processes.

EP12 How nurses analyze data to guide decisions regarding unit and department budget formulation, implementation, monitoring, and evaluation.

Interdisciplinary Care. Describe and demonstrate

EP13 How nurses have assumed leadership roles in interdisciplinary collaboration.

EP14 How the organization ensures the participation of nurses at all levels in interdisciplinary activities to develop policy and standards of care.

EP15 Interdisciplinary collaboration using continuous quality and process improvement.

EP16 Interdisciplinary collaboration across multiple settings to ensure the continuum of care.

EP17 Interdisciplinary collaboration to ensure that information systems and technology used for clinical care monitoring, documentation, and communication are integrated and evaluated.

EP18 Interdisciplinary collaboration to develop, implement, and evaluate a comprehensive set of patient education programs and resources within the organization.

Accountability, Competence, and Autonomy. Describe and demonstrate

EP19 That nurses have ready access to, and routinely use, current literature, professional standards, and other data sources to support autonomous practice.

EP20 That nurses at all levels routinely use self-appraisal performance review and peer review, including annual goal setting, for the assurance of competence and professional development.

EP21 The structure(s) and process(es) that support shared leadership/participative decision-making and promote nursing autonomy.

EP22 That nurses are accountable to resolve issues related to patient care or operational issues.

Ethics, Privacy, Security, and Confidentiality. Describe and demonstrate

EP23 How nurses use available resources, such as the *ANA Code of Ethics for Nurses* (American Nurses Association, 2001b), to address complex ethical issues. Provide examples from different practice settings.

EP24 How nurses have resolved issues related to patient privacy, security, and confidentiality.

Diversity and Workplace Advocacy. Describe and demonstrate

EP25 How the organization identifies and addresses disparities in the management of the healthcare needs of diverse patient populations. Include the role of the nurse.

EP26 How nurses use resources to meet the unique and individual needs of patients and families.

EP27 How the organization promotes a non-discriminatory climate for patients.

MAGNET DICTIONARY

autonomy
"Professional nurse autonomy implies the right to exercise clinical and organizational judgment within the context of an interdependent health care team and in accordance with the socially and legally granted freedom of the discipline" (MacDonald, 2002, as cited in Tranmer, 2005, p. 141). "Organizational autonomy is an environmental characteristic that involves nurses in the broader unit and hospital decision-making processes pertaining to patient care. Clinical autonomy and organizational autonomy or control over nursing practice are interactive concepts" (Hinshaw, 2002, p. 92-93).

competence
The Institute of Medicine (2003) defined professional competence as "the habitual and judicious use of communication, knowledge, technical skills, clinical reasoning, emotions, values, and reflection in daily practice for the benefit of the individuals and community being served."

EP28 The organizational structure(s) and process(es) that are in place to identify and manage problems related to incompetent, unsafe, or unprofessional conduct.

EP29 The organization's workplace advocacy initiatives for:
- Caregiver stress
- Diversity
- Rights
- Confidentiality

Culture of Safety. Describe and demonstrate

EP30 The structure(s) and process(es) used by the organization to improve workplace safety for nurses, based on recommendations such as the *ANA's Safe Patient Handling and Movement* (http://www.nursingworld.org/ MainMenuCategories/ANAPoliticalPower/Federal/Issues/SPHM.aspx).

EP30EO Two (2) workplace safety improvements for nurses that resulted from the structure(s) and process(es) in EP30.

EP31 How the organization uses a facility-wide approach for proactive risk assessment and error management.

EP32 The nursing structure(s) and process(es) that support a culture of patient safety.

EP32EO That nursing-sensitive indicator data aggregated at the organization or unit level outperform the mean, median or other benchmark statistic of the national database used. Provide analysis and evaluation of data related to patient falls, nosocomial pressure ulcer prevalence and/or incidence, and two (2) of the following:
- Blood stream infections
- Urinary tract infections
- Ventilator-associated pneumonia
- Restraint use
- Pediatric IV infiltrations
- Other specialty-specific nationally benchmarked indicators (use only for units for which the above do not apply)

Quality Care Monitoring and Improvement. Describe and demonstrate

EP33 The structure(s) and process(es) used by the organization to allocate and/or reallocate resources to monitor and improve the quality of nursing, and total patient care. The nurse has responsibility for ensuring the coordination of care among other disciplines and support staff.

EP33EO How the allocation and/or reallocation of resources improved the quality of nursing care.

EP34 How nurse leaders ensure the dissemination of comprehensive quality data to direct-care nurses.

EP35 The structure(s) and process(es) used to identify significant findings and trends in overall patient satisfaction with nursing as compared to benchmarked sources.

EP35EO That patient satisfaction data aggregated at the organization or unit level outperform the mean, median or other benchmark statistic of the national database used. Provide analysis and evaluation of data and resultant action plans related to patient satisfaction with nursing addressing four (4) of the following:
- Pain
- Education
- Courtesy and respect from nurses
- Careful listening by nurses
- Response time
- Other nurse-related national survey questions

INITIAL APPLICATION

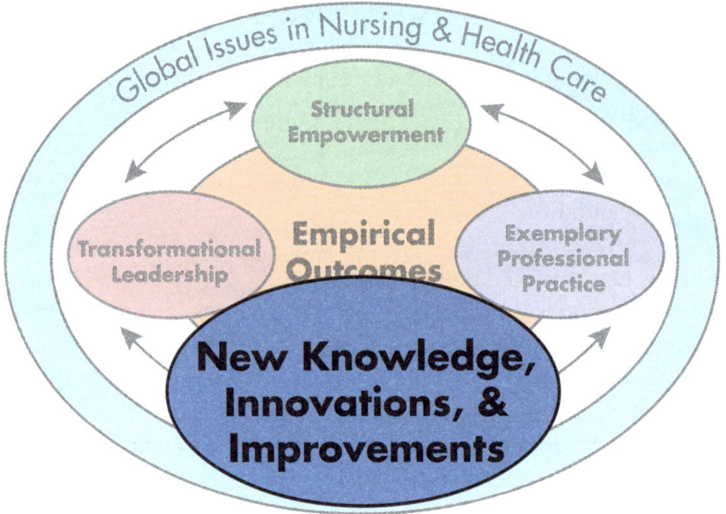

FORCES OF MAGNETISM
- QUALITY OF CARE: RESEARCH AND EVIDENCE-BASED PRACTICE
- QUALITY IMPROVEMENT

INITIAL APPLICATION

IV. New Knowledge, Innovations, and Improvements (NK)

Magnet organizations conscientiously integrate evidence-based practice and research into clinical and operational processes. Nurses are educated about evidence-based practice and research, enabling them to appropriately explore the safest and best practices for their patients and practice environment, and to generate new knowledge. Published research is systematically evaluated and used. Nurses serve on the board that reviews proposals for research, and knowledge gained through research is disseminated to the community of nurses.

Organizations achieving Magnet recognition possess established and evolving programs related to evidence-based practices and research programs. Infrastructures and resources are in place to support the advancement of evidence-based practices and research in all clinical settings. Targets for research productivity are set with participation and leadership in a multitude of research activities within the framework of the practice site.

Innovations in patient care, nursing, and the practice environment are the hallmark of organizations receiving Magnet recognition. Establishing new ways of achieving high-quality, effective, and efficient care is the outcome of transformational leadership, empowering structures and processes, and exemplary professional practice in nursing.

Sources of Evidence

Research. Describe and demonstrate

NK1   That nurses at all levels evaluate and use published research findings in their practice.

NK2   Consistent membership and involvement by at least one (1) nurse in the governing body responsible for the protection of human subjects in research, and that a nurse votes on nursing-related protocols.

NK3   That direct-care nurses support the human rights of participants in research protocols.

NK4   The structure(s) and process(es) used by the organization to develop, expand, and/or advance nursing research.

NK4E0   Nursing research studies from the past 2 years, ongoing or completed, generated from the structure(s) and process(es) in NK4. Provide a table including:
- Study title
- Study status
- Principal investigator name(s)
- Principal investigator credential(s)
- Role(s) of nurses in the study
- Study scope (internal to a single organization, multiple organizations within a system, independent organizations collaboratively)
- Study type (replication—yes or no; qualitative, quantitative, or both)

Select one (1) completed research study and respond to the four (4) criteria listed in the EO guidelines provided in this chapter (page 34).

NK5   How the organization disseminates knowledge generated through nursing research to internal and external audiences.

Evidence-Based Practice. Describe and demonstrate

NK6   The structure(s) and process(es) used to evaluate existing nursing practice, based on evidence.

NK7   The structure(s) and process(es) used to translate new knowledge into nursing practice.

NK7EO   How translation of new knowledge into nursing practice has affected patient outcomes.

Innovation. Describe and demonstrate

NK8   Innovations in nursing practice.

NK9   The structure(s) and process(es) by which nurses are involved with the evaluation and allocation of technology and information systems to support practice, or nurses' participation in architecture and space design to support practice.

NK9EO   An improvement in practice due to nurse involvement in technology and information system decision-making, or due to nurses' participation in architecture and space design.

MAGNET DICTIONARY

nursing research
A systematic search for knowledge about issues of importance to the nursing profession (Polit and Hungler, 1995).

INITIAL APPLICATION

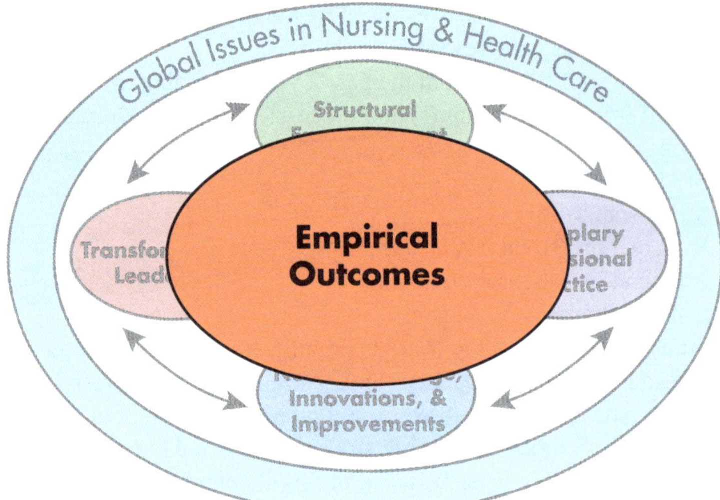

FORCES OF MAGNETISM
• QUALITY CARE

MAGNET DICTIONARY

outcomes
Quantitative and qualitative evidence related to the impact of structure and process on the patient, nursing workforce, organization, and consumer. These outcomes are dynamic; measurable; and may be reported at an individual unit, department, population, or organizational level. Donabedian (1980) defined *outcomes* as the "changes (desirable or undesirable) in individuals and populations that can be attributed to health care" (see 2003, p. 46).

V. Empirical Outcomes (EO)

Nursing makes an essential contribution to patient, nursing workforce, organizational, and consumer outcomes. The empirical measurement of quality outcomes related to nursing leadership and clinical practice in Magnet organizations is imperative. Throughout this *Manual,* in each of the other model components, the Empirical Outcomes (EO) are requested as Sources of Evidence.

Display of data using graphs and charts is an excellent way to illustrate outcomes. When documenting evidence in response to an EO, unless already addressed in the associated Source of Evidence, include the following information in the response:
• Describe the purpose and the background.
• Describe how the work was done (methods or approach).
• Discuss who (CNO, staff RNs, CFO, APRNs, pharmacists, physicians, etc.) was involved and what units participated.
• Describe the measurement used to evaluate the outcomes and the impact (show results and significance of the results).

The relationships among the structure and processes of care and associated outcomes need to be continually assessed and monitored. EOs focus on the results and the differences that can be demonstrated based on the application of sound structure and processes in the healthcare team, organization, and systems of care.

Outcomes are dynamic and define areas of both improved performance and those requiring additional effort to achieve improvement. Organizations must establish baselines for measures and track progress over time compared to the baseline and national benchmarks. Magnet organizations are expected to serve as mentors and lead the way in the provision of quality patient care and the creation of environments that contribute to the well-being of the workforce and the community at large.

See Chapter 6 for site visit preparation and activities.

5

Evidence Submission for Redesignating Applicants

This section describes the redesignation expectations for each of the five (5) Model components. Redesignating organizations submit written documentation on a subset of the Sources of Evidence. A greater emphasis is placed on demonstrating excellence through quality outcomes and innovative practice.

As Magnet organizations mature, and structure and processes are hardwired, a greater emphasis will be placed on outcomes at the time of redesignation. To sustain Magnet designation, many Magnet hospitals seek to maintain stability in structures and processes that have contributed to past success. However, only seeking stability can interfere with innovation intended to achieve cutting-edge performance. To achieve this support for innovation, the Commission on Magnet Recognition (COM) shifted the weighting of the scores of each of the Model components (see Table 6) by weighting the New Knowledge and Empirical Outcomes sections higher (highlighted in gold) for organizations seeking redesignation.

TABLE 6. WEIGHT OF THE COMPONENTS OF THE MAGNET MODEL

NEW APPLICANTS	REDESIGNATING MAGNETS
Transformational Leadership	Transformational Leadership
Structural Empowerment	Structural Empowerment
Exemplary Professional Practice	Exemplary Professional Practice
New Knowledge, Innovations, and Improvements	New Knowledge, Innovations, and Improvements
Empirical Outcomes	Empirical Outcomes

Key: Gold highlights represent more heavily-weighted components.

Table 7 depicts the labeling convention used to refer to the Sources of Evidence by Magnet Model component (e.g., TL4 or TL4EO). The Sources of Evidence are further subcategorized for easy understanding (e.g., *Strategic Planning, Advocacy and Influence, and Visibility and Accessibility*).

TABLE 7. REFERENCE LABELS OF THE SOURCES OF EVIDENCE

LABEL	MODEL COMPONENT	SOURCE NUMBER	OUTCOME IDENTIFIER
TL	Transformational Leadership	TL1, TL2, etc.	TL3EO, etc
SE	Structural Empowerment	SE1, SE2, etc.	SE2EO, etc.
EP	Exemplary Professional Practice	EP1, EP2, etc.	EP1EO, etc.
NK	New Knowledge, Innovations, and Improvements	NK1, NK2, etc.	NK4EO, etc.
EO	Empirical Outcomes		

Note that the EO sources are embedded as part of the other four (4) Model components. Writing guidelines for EOs are described on page 52.

ORGANIZATIONAL OVERVIEW FOR REDESIGNATION

The following documents must be present for the appraisers to score the Sources of Evidence. The Sources of Evidence that correlate with an Organizational Overview item for scoring are indicated in parentheses following the item. See the web site at http://www.nursecredentialing.org/Magnet/ApplicationProcess/MagnetReconitionProgramDownloadForms.aspx for required tables.

Contextual Information
1. A description of the applicant organization in terms of:
    - Mission
    - Vision
    - Values
    - History
    - Geographical location
    - Services provided
    - Number of licensed beds
    - Total RN full-time equivalents
    - Population(s) served

Include an ethnic profile of the nursing staff, client population, and community served.

2. The current chief nursing officer's (CNO) job description and curriculum vitae.

Transformational Leadership
3. Copies of the most recent annual reports, quality and strategic plans for the organization and nursing services. These can be formal documents or less formal methods used to inform the staff of activities related to the strategic plan. (TL1)

4. A budget summary for the most recent fiscal year, actual to budget, for nursing education, conference attendance, and research. (TL2 & EP12)

5. The administrative and nursing organizational chart(s). Describe the CNO's structural and operational relationships to all areas in which nursing is practiced. (TL4)

6. A table of nurse executives, nurse managers, and supervisors and their:
   - Credentials;
   - Earned professional certification(s);
   - Professional organization memberships, activities, and offices held; and
   - Professional development programs and formal academic education attended during the 24 months prior to documentation submission.

Structural Empowerment

7. A table that displays direct-care nurses' participation in professional organizations/associations and activities at the local, state, national, and/or international levels. Include office(s) held. (SE2)

8. The policies and procedures that govern/guide professional development programs, such as tuition reimbursement; access to web-based education; and participation in local, regional, national, and international conferences/meetings. (SE3, SE4, & SE5)

9. The assessment for the continuing education needs of nurses at all levels and settings, and the related implementation plan. (SE5)

10. A list of the continuing education programs (classroom and/or electronic) and the number of nurses completing each during the past 24 months. Do not include orientation activities or in-service education. Include programs covering each of the following topics: (SE5)
    - Research, including protection of human subjects
    - Evidence-based practice
    - Application of ethical principles
    - *ANA Bill of Rights for Nurses* (American Nurses Association, 2001a)
    - Professional standards of practice and performance
    - Cultural competence
    - Data and information analysis competencies
    - Quality improvement
    - Leadership
    - Nurse Practice Act (or similar document for international applicants)
    - Patient privacy, security, and confidentiality
    - Regulatory requirements

Exemplary Professional Practice

11. Describe the Professional Practice Model(s) and the Care Delivery System(s) in use in the organization. The *Professional Practice Model* is a schematic description of a theory, phenomenon, or system that depicts how nurses practice, collaborate, communicate, and develop professionally. A *Care Delivery System* delineates nurses' authority and accountability for clinical decision-making and outcomes. If possible, provide a depiction of each model. (EP1, EP1EO, EP3, EP4, EP7, & EP12)

12. Unit-based, nationally benchmarked nurse satisfaction or engagement data for a 2- or 3-year period to include data from the most recent two (2) survey cycles. If available, include the levels of statistical significance as compared to the benchmark. Include a graphic display of the data that clearly identifies benchmarks. (EP3)

13. For U.S. applicants, case mix index information, by unit, service or product line, for each of the two (2) 1-year periods immediately preceding the submission of written documentation. If this is not feasible, explain why. (EP8)

14. The actual to budgeted direct Nursing Care Hours/Patient Day (HPPD) or hours per workload index by unit for each of the two (2) 1-year periods immediately preceding the submission of written documentation. (EP11)

15. A table of the interdisciplinary committees and task forces at the organizational level, a description of each one's purpose, and guidelines for decision-making. Include nurse membership and role on the committee. Indicate each nurse's work unit(s) and role(s) in the organization. (EP13 & EP16)

16. Access to the state's Nurse Practice Act. It is sufficient to provide the web address of this document after validating that the most current version of the act is available on the web site. If this is not the case, provide a hard copy of the most current version of the act.

17. Performance appraisal tools, if used, and all associated peer evaluation tools for staff nurses and nurse leaders. Include frequency of evaluation. If the organization uses multiple versions of these tools, provide a representative sample for all levels of nurses. (EP20)

18. A description of the process by which the CNO or his or her designeé participates in credentialing, privileging, and evaluating advanced-practice nurses. Include the frequency of re-privileging.

19. The policies and procedures that address patient ethical issues/needs. Describe the leadership of nurses in developing and participating in these programs. (EP23)

20. The policies and procedures that permit and encourage nurses to confidentially express their concerns about their professional practice environment without retribution. (EP28)

21. The policies and procedures that address the identification and management of problems related to incompetent, unsafe, or unprofessional practice or conduct. (EP28)

22. The policies and procedures regarding interdisciplinary conflict. (EP29)

23. Nursing-sensitive indicator data related to patient outcomes for a 2-year period. If available, include the levels of statistical significance as compared to the benchmark. Data at the unit level by measure must be submitted on patient falls, nosocomial pressure ulcer incidence and/or prevalence, along with two (2) (the same data sets as used in response to EP32EO) of the following:
    - Blood stream infections
    - Urinary tract infections
    - Ventilator-associated pneumonia
    - Restraint use
    - Pediatric IV infiltrations
    - Other specialty-specific nationally benchmarked indicators

Include a graphic display of the data that clearly identifies benchmarks. List all external databases used to benchmark your performance. (EP32) *Note*: By 2012, organizations must provide unit-level data on all applicable indicators listed above.

24. Nursing-sensitive indicator data related to nurse work-related injuries such as needle sticks, musculoskeletal injuries, and exposures (e.g., laser, chemicals, toxins, infectious agents). (EP30)

25. A description of the infrastructure, the organizational committees, and decision-making bodies specifically designed to oversee the quality of patient care. (EP33)

26. Patient satisfaction data at the unit level by measure for a 2-year period, including statistical levels of significance. Include a graphic display of the data that clearly identifies benchmarks. (EP35)

New Knowledge, Innovations, and Improvements

27. The institution's policies, procedures (including Institutional Review Board), and processes that protect the rights of participants in research. (NK2)

28. The credentials or related experience of all external experts and other resources used to develop and/or improve the infrastructures, capacities, and processes for evidence-based practice and research. (NK4 & NK4EO)

COMPONENTS AND SOURCES OF EVIDENCE

This section presents the conceptual definitions for the five (5) components and lists the Magnet program Sources of Evidence, which are represented by initials for their respective component (e.g., TL5 for Source of Evidence 5 under Transformational Leadership). Each EO, for documentation purposes, is included with its associated component (e.g., SE2EO for the EO associated with Source of Evidence 2 under Structural Empowerment). The Sources of Evidence are further sub-categorized for easy understanding (e.g., *Strategic Planning, Advocacy and Influence, and Visibility and Accessibility*).

FORCES OF MAGNETISM
- QUALITY OF NURSING LEADERSHIP
- MANAGEMENT STYLE

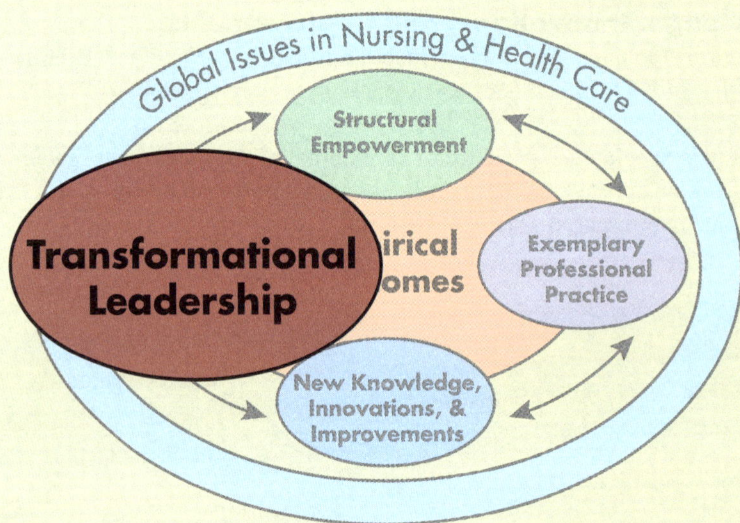

I. Transformational Leadership (TL)

The CNO in a Magnet organization is a knowledgeable, transformational leader who develops a strong vision and well-articulated philosophy, Professional Practice Model, and strategic and quality plans in leading nursing services. The transformational CNO communicates expectations, develops leaders, and evolves the organization to meet current and anticipated needs and strategic priorities. Nursing leaders at all levels of the organization convey a strong sense of advocacy and support on behalf of staff and patients.

The CNO must be strategically positioned within the organization to effectively influence other executive stakeholders, including the board of directors/trustees. Strategic positioning is imperative to achieving the level of influence required to lead others both operationally and during periods of change management due to internal or external factors. Executive-level nursing leaders serve at the executive level of the organization, with the CNO typically reporting to the chief executive officer.

The nursing organization must be continually assessed, and appropriate strategic and quality plans for nursing and patient care developed that are congruent with those of the organization. The CNO must secure adequate resources to implement these plans and engage in interdisciplinary efforts to accomplish this work.

Wherever nursing is practiced, the CNO must develop structures, processes, and expectations for staff nurse input and involvement throughout the organization. Mechanisms must be implemented for evidence-based practice to evolve and for innovation to flourish. The CNO should be seen as an executive leader and a nursing advocate and perceived as leading nursing practice and patient care. The CNO is visible, accessible, and communicates effectively in an environment of mutual respect. As a result, nurses throughout the organization should perceive that their voices are heard, their input valued, and their practice supported.

Sources of Evidence

Strategic Planning. Describe and demonstrate

TL1	How nursing's mission, vision, values, and strategic and quality plans reflect the organization's current and anticipated strategic priorities.
TL2	How nurses at every level—CNO, nurse administrators, and direct-care nurses—advocate for resources, including fiscal and technology resources, to support unit/division goals.
TL3	The strategic planning structure(s) and process(es) used by nursing to improve the healthcare system's: • Effectiveness and • Efficiency.
TL3EO	The outcome(s) that resulted from the planning described in TL3.

Advocacy and Influence. Describe and demonstrate

TL4	The process(es) that enable the CNO to influence organization-wide changes.
TL4EO	One (1) CNO-influenced organization-wide change.
TL5	How nurse leaders guide the transition during periods of planned or unplanned change.
TL7	How nurse leaders value, encourage, recognize/reward, and implement innovation.

Visibility, Accessibility, and Communication. Describe and demonstrate

TL10	How nurse leaders use input from direct care nurses to improve the work environment and patient care.
TL10EO	Changes in the work environment and patient care based on input from the direct-care nurses.

FORCES OF MAGNETISM
- ORGANIZATIONAL STRUCTURE
- PERSONNEL POLICIES AND PROGRAMS
- COMMUNITY AND THE HEALTHCARE ORGANIZATION
- IMAGE OF NURSING
- PROFESSIONAL DEVELOPMENT

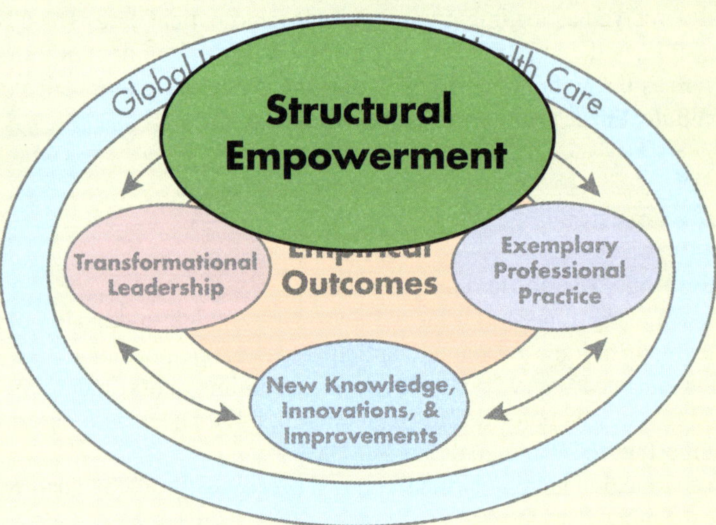

II. Structural Empowerment (SE)

Magnet structural environments are generally flat, flexible, and decentralized. Nurses throughout the organization are involved in self-governance and decision-making structures and processes that establish standards of practice and address issues of concern. The flow of information and decision-making is bi-directional and horizontal between and among professional nurses at the bedside, the leadership team, and the CNO. The CNO serves on the highest-level councils and/or committees. Nurse leaders throughout the organization also serve on committees and task forces that address excellence in patient care and the safe, efficient, and effective operation of the organization.

The healthcare organization promotes relationships among all types of community organizations to develop strong partnerships to improve patient outcomes and the health of the communities they serve. Magnet nurses extend their influence to professional and community groups, advancing the nursing profession and supporting organizational goals and personal and professional growth and development.

The organization uses multiple strategies to establish structures, systematic and equitable processes, and expectations that support lifelong professional learning, role development, and career advancement. Relationships are established throughout the organization and with the community to encourage educational advancement.

Nurse contributions to the organization and community are recognized for their positive effect on patients and families. Nurses are acknowledged in various and substantive ways for these accomplishments, enhancing the image of nursing in the community.

Sources of Evidence

Professional Engagement. Describe and demonstrate

SE1   The structure(s) and process(es) that enable nurses from all settings and roles to actively participate in organizational decision-making groups such as committees, councils, and task forces.

SE1EO   Two (2) improvements in different practice settings because of nurse involvement in organizational decision-making groups such as committees, councils, and task forces.

SE2   The structure(s) and process(es) that enable nurses at all levels to participate in professional nursing organizations at the local, state, and national levels. Include international participation, if any.

SE2EO   Two (2) improvements in different practice settings that occurred because of nurse involvement in a professional nursing organization(s).

Commitment to Professional Development. Describe and demonstrate

SE3   How the organization sets expectations and supports nurses at all levels who seek additional formal nursing education (e.g., baccalaureate, master's, doctoral degrees).

SE3EO   That the organization has met goals for improvement in formal education. Graphically summarize at least 2 years of data to display changes over time.

SE4   How the organization sets goals and supports professional development and professional certification, such as tuition/registration reimbursement and participation in external local, regional, national, and international conferences or meetings.

SE4EO   That the organization has met goals for improvement in professional certification. Graphically summarize at least 2 years of data to display changes over time. Include participation of nurses in all specialties.

SE5   The structure(s) and process(es) used by nursing to develop and provide continuing education programs for nurses at all levels and settings. Include how the organization provides onsite internal electronic and classroom methods. Do not include orientation.

SE5EO   The effectiveness of two (2) educational programs provided in SE5.

Commitment to Community Involvement. Describe and demonstrate

SE11   The structure(s) and process(es) used to identify and allocate resources for affiliations with schools of nursing, consortiums, or community outreach programs.

SE11EO   The result(s) of the affiliations with schools of nursing, consortiums, or community outreach programs described in SE11.

SE13   How the organization or nursing addresses the healthcare needs of the community by establishing partnerships.

Recognition of Nursing. Describe and demonstrate

SE15   That the nursing community and the community at large (e.g., local, state, national, international) recognize the value of nursing in the organization.

FORCES OF MAGNETISM
- PROFESSIONAL MODELS OF CARE
- CONSULTATION AND RESOURCES
- AUTONOMY
- NURSES AS TEACHERS
- INTERDISCIPLINARY RELATIONSHIPS
- QUALITY OF CARE: ETHICS, PATIENT SAFETY AND QUALITY INFRASTRUCTURE
- QUALITY IMPROVEMENT

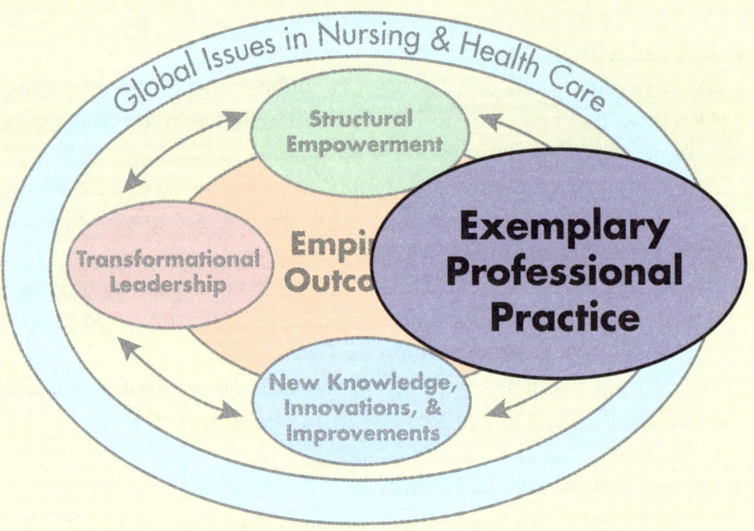

III. Exemplary Professional Practice (EP)

A Professional Practice Model is the overarching conceptual framework for nurses, nursing care, and interdisciplinary patient care. It is a schematic description of a system, theory, or phenomenon that depicts how nurses practice, collaborate, communicate, and develop professionally to provide the highest quality care for those served by the organization (e.g., patients, families, community). The Professional Practice Model illustrates the alignment and integration of nursing practice with the mission, vision, philosophy, and values that nursing has adapted. Magnet hospitals take the lead in research efforts to create and test models of professional practice for nurses.

The Care Delivery System is integrated within the Professional Practice Model and promotes continuous, consistent, efficient, and accountable delivery of nursing care. The Care Delivery System is adapted to regulatory considerations and describes the manner in which care is delivered, skill set required, context of care, and expected outcomes of care. Nurses create patient care delivery systems that delineate the nurses' authority and accountability for clinical decision-making and outcomes. At the organizational level, nurse leaders ensure that care is patient/family centered.

Exemplary professional practice is evident in Magnet hospitals. Nurses have significant control over staffing and scheduling processes and work in collaboration with interdisciplinary partners to achieve high-quality patient outcomes.

Interdisciplinary collaboration is evident with clear expectations and direction to all practicing nurses about the importance of partnerships with patients and families, and with the disciplines of medicine, pharmacy, nutrition, rehabilitation, social work, psychology, and other professions to ensure a comprehensive care plan. Collegial working relationships within and among the disciplines are valued by the organization and its employees. Mutual respect is based on the premise that all members of the healthcare team make essential and meaningful contributions in the achievement of clinical outcomes. Conflict management strategies are in place and used effectively, when indicated.

The autonomous nurse makes judgments about how to provide care based on the unique needs and attributes of the patient and family. The knowledge, skills, and resources that have been identified by the nursing staff as necessary to practice are consistently available in the practice environment. These resources form the basis of the Care Delivery System. Competency assessment and peer evaluation ensures that the nurse bases care delivery decisions on current evidence about safe and ethical practice using the nursing process.

Attention is given to achieving equity in care. Workplace advocacy initiatives address ethical issues and the privacy, security, and confidentiality of patients and staff.

The achievement of exemplary professional practice is grounded by a culture of safety, quality monitoring, and quality improvement. Nurses collaborate with other disciplines to ensure that care is comprehensive, coordinated, and monitored for effectiveness through the quality improvement model. Nurses participate in safety initiatives that incorporate national best practices. Sufficient resources are available to respond to safety initiatives and quality improvements for patients and employees.

Nurses at all levels analyze data and use national benchmarks to gain a comparative perspective about their performance and the care patients receive. Action plans are developed that lead to systematic improvements over time. Magnet hospital data demonstrate outcome measures that outperform the benchmark statistic of the national database used in patient and nursing-sensitive indicators the majority of the time.

Sources of Evidence

Professional Practice Model. Describe and demonstrate

EP1   How nurses develop, apply, evaluate, adapt, and modify the Professional Practice Model.

EP1EO   The result(s) of applying the Professional Practice Model. Include two (2) examples related to nursing practice, collaboration, communication, or professional development activities.

EP3   The structure(s) and process(es) that include direct-care nurse involvement in tracking and analyzing nurse satisfaction or engagement data.

EP3EO   That nurse satisfaction or engagement data aggregated at the organization or unit level outperform the mean, median or other benchmark statistic of the national database used. Include participation rates, analysis, and evaluation of the data.

Care Delivery System(s). Describe and demonstrate

EP4   That the structure(s) and process(es) of the Care Delivery System(s) involve the patient and/or his or her support system in the planning and delivery of care. Provide at least two (2) examples of a plan of care that included patient and/or family member involvement.

EP7   The structure(s) and process(es) used to engage internal experts and external consultants to improve care in the practice setting.

EP7EO   Two (2) improvements in the practice setting that occurred as a result of the use of internal experts or external consultants.

Staffing, Scheduling, and Budgeting Processes. Describe and demonstrate

EP8   How nurses use trended data to formulate the staffing plan and acquire necessary resources to assure consistent application of the Care Delivery System(s).

EP9   How direct-care nurses participate in staffing and scheduling processes.

EP11   How guidelines such as the *ANA Principles of Nurse Staffing* (American Nurses Association, 2005), standards for scheduling, delegation, and from nursing specialty organizations and/or state-mandated requirements are incorporated into staffing and scheduling processes.

EP12   How nurses analyze data to guide decisions regarding unit and department budget formulation, implementation, monitoring, and evaluation.

Interdisciplinary Care. Describe and demonstrate

EP13   How nurses have assumed leadership roles in interdisciplinary collaboration.

EP16   Interdisciplinary collaboration across multiple settings to ensure the continuum of care.

Accountability, Competence, and Autonomy. Describe and demonstrate

EP20   That nurses at all levels routinely use self-appraisal performance review and peer review, including annual goal setting, for the assurance of competence and professional development.

Ethics, Privacy, Security, and Confidentiality. Describe and demonstrate

EP23   How nurses use available resources, such as the *ANA Code of Ethics for Nurses* (American Nurses Association, 2001b), to address complex ethical issues. Provide examples from different practice settings.

Diversity and Workplace Advocacy. Describe and demonstrate

EP26   How nurses use resources to meet the unique and individual needs of patients and families.

EP28   The organizational structure(s) and process(es) that are in place to identify and manage problems related to incompetent, unsafe, or unprofessional conduct.

EP29   The organization's workplace advocacy initiatives for:
- Caregiver stress
- Diversity
- Rights
- Confidentiality

Culture of Safety. Describe and demonstrate

EP30   The structure(s) and process(es) used by the organization to improve workplace safety for nurses, based on recommendations such as the *ANA's Safe Patient Handling and Movement* (http://www.nursingworld.org/MainMenuCategories/ANAPoliticalPower/Federal/Issues/SPHM.aspx).

EP30EO   Two (2) workplace safety improvements for nurses that resulted from the structure(s) and process(es) in EP30.

EP31   How the organization uses a facility-wide approach for proactive risk assessment and error management.

EP32   The nursing structure(s) and process(es) that support a culture of patient safety.

EP32EO   That nursing-sensitive indicator data aggregated at the organization or unit level outperform the mean, median or other benchmark statistic of the national database used. Provide analysis and evaluation of data related to patient falls, nosocomial pressure ulcer prevalence and/or incidence, and two (2) of the following:
- Blood stream infections
- Urinary tract infections
- Ventilator-associated pneumonia
- Restraint use

- Pediatric IV infiltrations
- Other specialty-specific nationally benchmarked indicators
  (use only for units for which the above do not apply)

Quality Care Monitoring and Improvement. Describe and demonstrate

EP33 The structure(s) and process(es) used by the organization to allocate and/or reallocate resources to monitor and improve the quality of nursing, and total patient care. The nurse has responsibility for ensuring the coordination of care among other disciplines and support staff.

EP33EO How the allocation and/or reallocation of resources improved the quality of nursing care.

EP35 The structure(s) and process(es) used to identify significant findings and trends in overall patient satisfaction with nursing as compared to benchmarked sources.

EP35EO That patient satisfaction data aggregated at the organization or unit level outperform the mean, median or other benchmark statistic of the national database used. Provide analysis and evaluation of data and resultant action plans related to patient satisfaction addressing four (4) of the following:

- Pain
- Education
- Courtesy and respect from nurses
- Careful listening by nurses
- Response time
- Other nurse-related national survey questions

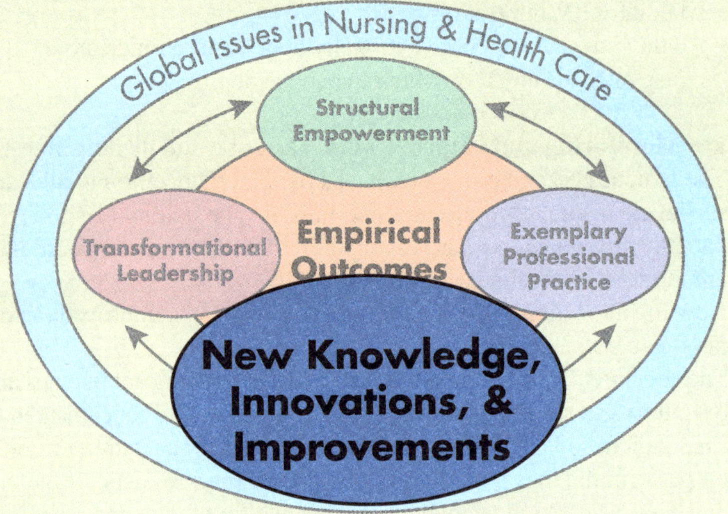

FORCES OF MAGNETISM
- QUALITY OF CARE: RESEARCH AND
  EVIDENCE-BASED PRACTICE
- QUALITY IMPROVEMENT

NOTE

A June 2008 survey of CNOs of ANCC Magnet-designated organizations revealed that, on average, the number of scholarly research studies ongoing or completed was at least one (1) per 100 licensed beds.

IV. New Knowledge, Innovations, and Improvements (NK)

Magnet organizations conscientiously integrate evidence-based practice and research into clinical and operational processes. Nurses are educated about evidence-based practice and research, enabling them to appropriately explore the safest and best practices for their patients and practice environment, and to generate new knowledge. Published research is systematically evaluated and used. Nurses serve on the board that reviews proposals for research, and knowledge gained through research is disseminated to the community of nurses.

Organizations achieving Magnet recognition possess established and evolving programs related to evidence-based practices and research programs. Infrastructures and resources are in place to support the advancement of evidence-based practices and research in all clinical settings. Targets for research productivity are set with participation and leadership in a multitude of research activities within the framework of the practice site.

Innovations in patient care, nursing, and the practice environment are the hallmark of organizations receiving Magnet recognition. Establishing new ways of achieving high-quality, effective, and efficient care is the outcome of transformational leadership, empowering structures and processes, and exemplary professional practice in nursing.

Sources of Evidence

Research. Describe and demonstrate
NK2   Consistent membership and involvement by at least one (1) nurse in the governing body responsible for the protection of human subjects in research, and that a nurse votes on nursing-related protocols.
NK4   The structure(s) and process(es) used by the organization to develop, expand, and/or advance nursing research.

NK4EO Nursing research studies from the past 2 years, ongoing or completed, generated from the structure(s) and process(es) in NK4. Provide a table including:
- Study title
- Study status
- Principal investigator name(s)
- Principal investigator credential(s)
- Role(s) of nurses in the study
- Study scope (internal to a single organization, multiple organizations within a system, independent organizations collaboratively)
- Study type (replication—yes or no; qualitative, quantitative, or both)

Select one (1) completed research study and respond to the four (4) criteria listed in the EO guidelines provided in this chapter (page 52).

Evidence-Based Practice. Describe and demonstrate

NK6 The structure(s) and process(es) used to evaluate existing nursing practice, based on evidence.

NK7 The structure(s) and process(es) used to translate new knowledge into nursing practice.

NK7EO How translation of new knowledge into nursing practice has affected patient outcomes.

Innovation. Describe and demonstrate

NK8 Innovations in nursing practice.

NK9 The structure(s) and process(es) by which nurses are involved with the evaluation and allocation of technology and information systems to support practice, or nurses' participation in architecture and space design to support practice.

NK9EO An improvement in practice due to nurse involvement in technology and information system decision-making, or due to nurses' participation in architecture and space design.

FORCES OF MAGNETISM
• QUALITY CARE

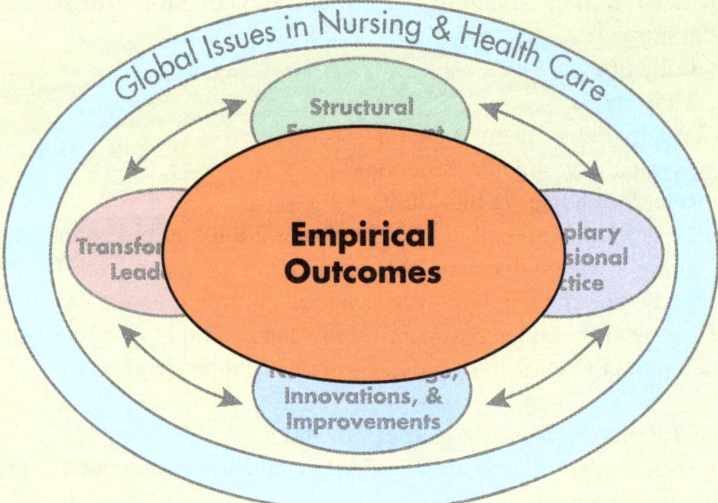

V. Empirical Outcomes (EO)

Nursing makes an essential contribution to patient, nursing workforce, organizational, and consumer outcomes. The empirical measurement of quality outcomes related to nursing leadership and clinical practice in Magnet organizations is imperative. Throughout this *Manual*, in each of the other model components, the Empirical Outcomes (EO) are requested as Sources of Evidence.

Display of data using graphs and charts is an excellent way to illustrate outcomes. When documenting evidence in response to an EO, unless already addressed in the associated Source of Evidence, include the following information in the response:
• Describe the purpose and the background.
• Describe how the work was done (methods or approach).
• Discuss who (CNO, staff RNs, CFO, APRNs, pharmacists, physicians, etc.) was involved and what units participated.
• Describe the measurement used to evaluate the outcomes and the impact (show results and significance of the results).

The relationships among the structure and processes of care and associated outcomes need to be continually assessed and monitored. EOs focus on the results and the differences that can be demonstrated based on the application of sound structure and processes in the healthcare team, organization, and systems of care.

Outcomes are dynamic and define areas of both improved performance and those requiring additional effort to achieve improvement. Organizations must establish baselines for measures and track progress over time compared to the baseline and national benchmarks. Magnet organizations are expected to serve as mentors and lead the way in the provision of quality patient care and the creation of environments that contribute to the well-being of the workforce and the community at large.

Site Visit Preparation and Activities

The Magnet site visit is an important evaluation activity for the healthcare organization. The goal of the visit is to verify, amplify, and clarify the contents of the written documentation and the presence of excellence in nursing throughout the organization. The site visit is the organization's opportunity to demonstrate the Magnet Model components are fully developed, disseminated, and enculturated in the organization.

SCHEDULING THE SITE VISIT AND PUBLIC NOTICE REQUIREMENTS

After determining an organization has met the requirements for a site visit, the assigned analyst from the Magnet Program Office will begin to negotiate the site visit dates between the applicant organization and the Magnet appraiser team. In general, the site visit can be scheduled no sooner than 40 business days after the decision is made, because the organization is required to post notices for public comment. The public notice will appear on the Magnet web site.

Employees, community stakeholders, and other interested parties may send communications about the applicant organization to the Magnet Program Office. Direct-care nurses from the applicant organization may participate in an on-line nurse survey located on the Magnet web site. The location of the web site will be identified in the public postings.

LENGTH OF THE SITE VISIT

The size of the organization, including inpatient and outpatient units and off-site service areas, determines the length of the site visit. Most visits are 3 days, plus or minus 1 day, depending on the number of licensed beds and distribution of the physical plants.

PAYMENT OF THE SITE VISIT FEE

- An invoice will be sent to the organization's chief nursing officer (CNO) when the site visit dates are confirmed.
- Mail the site visit fee, payable to ANCC *(not ANA)*, to:
American Nurses Credentialing Center, PO Box 79120, Baltimore, MD 21279-0120.
- If the site visit fee check is sent via FedEx, the address is:
SunTrust, Attention: Lock Box Services #79120, 1000 Stewart Avenue, Glen Burnie, MD 21061-3209.

PREPARATION OF THE SITE VISIT AGENDA

The Magnet team leader drafts the agenda for discussion with the Magnet program director and/or the CNO. The site visit agenda will include meetings with large and small groups and visits to the units and other areas where nurses work. Meetings with randomly selected direct-care nurses will occur. Once finalized, the agenda is open for modification during the site visit.

PREPARATION FOR THE SITE VISIT

Nurses should be able to comfortably talk about the programs, practices, and nursing outcomes within the organization. Preparation for the site visit will likely include some of the following:
- Random selection by the appraisers of direct-care nurses for group meetings
- Random selection by the appraisers of names of direct-care nurses and members of the leadership team for review of personnel files
- Visits with members of the community and area schools of nursing
- A meeting with labor union members, if applicable
- Review of current budget, nursing-sensitive indicators, nurse and patient satisfaction data, and advocacy department files reflecting reports related to nurses and nursing
- Identification of a room that is not monitored by the organization for the appraisers to use during the site visit

SITE VISIT ACTIVITIES

The appraisal team will meet with the CNO on each day of the site visit. This meeting is intended to confirm the agenda for the day, as well as address any concerns the team might have as it reviews documents, talks with staff, and visits units. This also is the time for the CNO to share his or her observation of the site visit and present any concerns for the appraisers to address.

The following will likely occur:
- Attendance will be taken at every meeting.
- Meetings will open with introductions by the team leader and appraiser team members, followed by introductions of the attendees.
- The meeting groups and clinical areas should not plan presentations, unless discussed in advance with the appraiser team leader.
- Direct-care nurses will serve as escorts and time keepers for the appraisers.
- The applicant is responsible for transporting the team to, from, and within the areas being evaluated.

- The appraisers will·visit most nursing units and departments that work closely with nursing.
- The role of management during the unit visits is indirect. When the appraisal team is engaged in clinical rounds, the nurse manager should not be present on the unit.
- Appraisers generally like to visit randomly-selected patients and families. Permission to do so must be obtained by the direct-care nursing staff.
- Appraisers may review a nurse's documentation, unit schedules, outcomes data, care plans, patient education materials, meeting minutes, and Internet search capabilities accessible by nurses.
- Gifts or mementos of any type should not be offered to the appraisers.
- Time is afforded in the agenda for members of the staff or community to "walk in" and speak with individual appraisers. A meeting room away from the administration offices is required. Requests for anonymity will always be honored.
- A thorough review of any concern from any source provided during the period of public comment will be conducted. Adjustments to the site visit agenda may be necessary in order to meet this responsibility.
- Although extremely rare, a site visit may be terminated for cause. Such an event would be coordinated by the Magnet Program Office, the appraiser team leader, and the CNO.

POST–SITE VISIT ACTIVITIES

The organization will receive an invitation to complete an on-line evaluation of the site visit. The feedback provided supports ANCC's commitment to continually evaluate the Magnet Recognition Program and to capitalize on recommendations for improvement. The information provided is not shared with the appraisal team or the Commission on Magnet Recognition (COM) until after the COM's decision is finalized.

Magnet Dictionary

accountability. The ethical concept of being answerable or responsible for one's actions. In nursing, personal accountability is the responsibility nurses have to themselves and to patients and public accountability is the responsibility nurses have to their employers and to society in general. "The primary goals of professional accountability in nursing are to maintain high standards of care and to protect the patient from harm. All nurses are accountable for the proper use of their knowledge and skills in the provision of care" (Farquharson, 2004, p. 311-312).

acute care. A healthcare organization in which care is delivered to hospitalized patients.

advanced-practice nurse (APRN). A registered nurse who has met advanced educational and clinical practice requirements beyond the 2–4 years of basic nursing education required of all RNs. Under this umbrella are four principal types of APRNs: nurse practitioners, certified nurse midwives, clinical nurse specialists, and certified registered nurse anesthetists.

all level of nurses. See *nurses at every level.*

ambulatory clinic. A facility in which people typically other than inpatients visit providers for treatment and/or health counseling.

autonomy. "Professional nurse autonomy implies the right to exercise clinical and organizational judgment within the context of an interdependent health care team and in accordance with the socially and legally granted freedom of the discipline" (MacDonald, 2002, as cited in Tranmer, 2005, p. 141). "Organizational autonomy is an environmental characteristic that involves nurses in the broader unit and hospital decision-making processes pertaining to patient care. Clinical autonomy and organizational autonomy or control over nursing practice are interactive concepts" (Hinshaw, 2002, p. 92-93).

beds. Operating beds for the care of patients staying 24 hours or more (category does not include bassinets).

benchmarking. Comparing data from the organization and other sources for the purpose of goal setting and performance measurements. To incorporate best practices into an organization's goal setting and performance measurement, benchmarking must use external as well as internal reference points. The contribution of data to benchmarking processes is an essential element of both research and quality improvement efforts in a variety of industries.

care delivery system. A system for the provision of care that delineates the nurses' authority and accountability for clinical decision-making and outcomes. The care delivery system is integrated with the practice model and promotes continuous, consistent, efficient, and accountable nursing care. The care delivery system is adapted to regulatory considerations and describes the context of care, the manner in which care is delivered, skill set required, and expected outcomes of care.

caregiver stress. Also called *moral distress*, a response experience when a decision-maker's ability to carry out a chosen ethical or moral action is thwarted by an individual, institutional, or societal constraint (Corley, Minick, Elswick, and Jacobs, 2005).

case mix index. A numerical score used in the United States as a descriptor at the organization level of the relative resource use for the *average* patient/client/resident. This use is computed using data on the characteristics and clinical needs of the patients/clients/residents served by the organization.

certification. A process by which a nongovernmental agency or association certifies that an individual licensed to practice a profession has met certain predetermined standards specified by that profession for specialty practice. Its purpose is to ensure various publics that an individual has mastered a body of knowledge and acquired skills in a particular specialty (American Nurses Association, 1979, p. 67). Certifications for ability to perform clinical interventions (e.g., Advanced Cardiac Life Support [ACLS], Basic Life Support [BLS], Neonatal Resuscitation Program [NRP], Pediatric Advanced Life Support [PALS]) are not included.

chief nursing officer (CNO). The nurse who participates in the management of healthcare services delivery by directing and coordinating the work of nursing and other personnel and representing nursing services. System applicants also should refer to Appendix D.

competence. The Institute of Medicine (2003) defined *professional competence* as "the habitual and judicious use of communication, knowledge, technical skills, clinical reasoning, emotions, values, and reflection in daily practice for the benefit of the individuals and community being served" (p. 24).

complaint. A written statement expressing dissatisfaction with, for example, service, practice, or professionalism. In contrast, a grievance is a formal complaint filed for resolution with a grievance system or process.

continuing education. Systematic professional learning experiences designed to augment the knowledge, skills, and attitudes of nurses' contributions to quality health care and their pursuit of professional career goals.

direct-care nurse. The nurse providing care directly to patients, excluding the nurse manager and nurse executive. (However, in some settings, the nurse manager does spend a portion of her or his work hours providing direct patient care.) Direct-care activities can be reflected as partial full-time equivalents (FTEs).

domain. A meaningful set of related concepts or indicators.

enculturation. A term synonymous with *socialization*, emphasizing that individuals have to constantly learn and use, both formally and informally, the prescribed patterns of cultural behavior in order to become full members of a culture or subculture. It is distinct from *acculturation*, which is synonymous with *assimilation*, a process by which an outsider/group becomes indistinguishably integrated into the dominant society (Scott and Marshall, 2005).

entity. A stand-alone group, whether or not within a system, whose nursing is governed by a CNO or a designated RN executive leader as identified in this glossary and whether or not separately legally established as a for-profit or non-profit, corporation, association, sole proprietorship, or partnership.

evidence-based practice (EBP). The conscientious use/integration of the best research evidence with clinical expertise and patient preferences in nursing practice (adapted from Sackett et al., 2000). EBP is a science-to-service model of engagement of critical thinking to apply research-based evidence (scientific knowledge) and practice-based evidence (art of nursing) within the context of patient values to deliver quality, cost-sensitive care. It is distinguished from *practice-based evidence (PBE)*, a practice-to-science model in which data are derived from interventions thought to be effective but for which empirical evidence is lacking. Providers are engaged in data collection, analysis, and synthesis to inform practice.

hospital system. The American Hospital Association (2007) defines *system* as "either a multihospital or a diversified single hospital system. A *multihospital system* is two or more hospitals owned, leased, sponsored, or contract managed by a central organization. *Single, freestanding* hospitals may be categorized as a system by bringing into membership three or more, and at least 25%, of their owned or leased non-hospital preacute or postacute healthcare organizations. System affiliation does not preclude network participation" (emphasis added).

hours per patient day (HPPD). Nursing care hours; direct hours of nursing care that are *patient* related, including nursing activities that occur away from the patient (e.g., care coordination, documentation time, treatment planning). This category does *not* include indirect hours, nonproductive time, or all-paid hours (e.g., vacation, sick time, orientation, education leave) and does *not* include committee time if the staff person is replaced by another direct caregiver. HPPD is calculated by the total number of direct RN nursing care hours divided by the patient/resident/client census for the same period.

innovation. "*Innovation* in service delivery and organization [is] a novel set of behaviors, routines, and ways of working that are directed at improving health outcomes, administrative efficiency, cost effectiveness, or users' experience and that are implemented by planned and coordinated actions" (Greenhalgh, 2004, emphasis added).

in-service education. Learning experiences provided in the work setting for the purpose of assisting staff members in performing their assigned functions in that particular agency or institution (American Nurses Association, 2000, p. 24).

Institutional Review Board (IRB). An independent committee comprised of scientific, non-scientific, and non-affiliated members established according to the requirements of U.S. federal regulations. Any board, committee, or other group formally designated by an organization to review research involving humans as participants, to approve the initiation of and conduct periodic review of such research. The term includes, but is not limited to, Institutional Review Boards, Investigational Review Boards, Central Review Boards, Independent Review Boards, and Cooperative Research Boards (U.S. Department of Health and Human Services, n.d., [45 CFR §46.402(g)] [21 CFR §50.3(i)]).

interdisciplinary. Reliant on the overlapping skills and knowledge of each team member and discipline, resulting in synergistic effects in which outcomes are improved and more comprehensive than the simple aggregation of any team member's individual efforts.

licensure/registration. The process of granting permission to engage in a specified activity or to perform a specified act. Permission generally is granted following confirmation of knowledge and abilities as evidenced by written, verbal, and/or demonstrated competencies in the performance or engagement of the specified activity or activities.

long-term care. A healthcare organization in which elderly and frail individuals reside.

multidisciplinary. Reliant on each team member or discipline contributing discipline-specific skills.

national certification. See *certification*.

National Labor Relations Board (NLRB). In the United States, the organization established to mediate and adjudicate collective-bargaining disputes regarding employment issues. See www.nlrb.gov.

new graduate. A nurse in first employment following completion of registered nurse education in the United States.

nurse. Generically, the registered professional nurse.

nurse administrator. A registered nurse whose primary responsibility is the management of healthcare services delivery and who represents nursing. For the purposes of this document, the two levels of nurse administrators are those of the *nurse executive* and the *nurse manager* (see entries below).

nurse engagement. A positive emotional connection to a nurses's work. Engagement as defined by Schaufeli, Salanova, González-romá, and Bakker (2002) is characterized by three dimensions: vigor, dedication, and absorption.

nurse leader. A nurse who participates in decision-making bodies and/or has a leadership role.

nurse manager. A Registered Nurse with 24 hour/7 day accountability for the overall supervision of all Registered Nurses and other healthcare providers who deliver nursing care in an inpatient or outpatient area. The Nurse Manager is typically responsible for recruitment and retention, performance review, and professional development; involved in the budget formulation process and quality outcomes; and helps to plan for, organize, and lead the delivery of nursing care for a designated patient care area.

Nurse Practice Act. The basic enabling law in states and territories within the United States for licensure and definition of nursing practice in the jurisdiction of the legislative body establishing the act. It defines who may practice nursing and, to some extent, how nursing will be practiced in the jurisdiction.

nurses at every level. This phrase is used when it is important that direct-care nurses and nurses in every role, not solely nurse managers and nurse administrators, participate in decision-making bodies.

nurse satisfaction. Job satisfaction expressed by nurses working in hospital settings as determined by scaled responses to a uniform series of questions designed to elicit nursing staff attitudes toward specific aspects of their employment situation.

nursing research. A systematic search for knowledge about issues of importance to the nursing profession (Polit and Hungler, 1995).

nursing-sensitive indicators. "Measures and indicators that reflect the impact of nursing actions on outcomes" (American Nurses Association, 2004, p. 25).

organization. A stand-alone structure within an entity; the term can by used interchangeably with *setting* where appropriate or necessary.

outcomes. Quantitative and qualitative evidence related to the impact of structure and process on the patient, nursing workforce, organization, and consumer. These outcomes are dynamic; measurable; and may be reported at an individual unit, department, population, or organizational level. Donabedian (1980) defined *outcomes* as the "changes (desirable or undesirable) in individuals and populations that can be attributed to health care" (see 2003, p. 46).

patient. A healthcare consumer across the variety of settings; he or she might variously be called a *patient*, *client*, or *resident*.

patient falls. An unplanned descent to the floor, either with or without injury to the patient/resident/client. Calculated by the total number of patient falls times 1,000 divided by total number of patient days.

patient overall satisfaction. Patient opinion of the care received during the hospital stay as determined by scaled responses to a uniform series of questions designed to elicit patient views about global aspects of care.

patient satisfaction with educational information. Patient opinion of nursing staff efforts to educate about condition and care requirements as determined by scaled responses to a uniform series of questions designed to elicit patient views about specific aspects of education activities.

patient satisfaction with nursing care. Patient opinion of care received from nursing staff during the hospital stay as determined by scaled responses to a uniform series of questions designed to elicit patient views about components of nursing care services.

patient satisfaction with pain management. Patient opinion of how well nursing staff managed pain as determined by scaled responses to a uniform series of questions designed to elicit patient views about specific aspects of pain management.

peer evaluation. Peer-provided components of an annual evaluation or performance appraisal, which may or may not include peer review, by which registered nurses assess and judge the performance of professional peers (i.e., registered nurses with similar roles and education, clinical expertise, and level of licensure) against predetermined standards. The peer review process stimulates professionalism through increased accountability and promotes self-regulation of practice.

pressure ulcer occurrence. Any lesion caused by pressure resulting in damage of underlying tissues. Other terms used to indicate this condition include *bed sores* and *decubitus ulcers*.

pressure ulcer prevalence. Calculated as the total number of decubitus ulcers (Grade I–IV) times 1,000 divided by total number of patient days.

process. The actions involving the delivery of nursing and healthcare services to patients, including practices that are safe and ethical, autonomous, evidence- based, and focused on quality improvement. Donabedian (1980) defined process as the activities constituting health care, "including diagnosis, treatment, rehabilitation, prevention, and patient education—usually carried out by professional personnel, but also including other contributions to care, particularly by patients and their families" (see 2003, p. 46).

professional organization. Professional bodies, which may be known as *organizations*, *associations*, or *societies*, that usually have the purpose of advancing a profession and protecting the public interest. Many professional organizations include voluntary certification processes among their functions as a vehicle to verify that members meet certain prespecified standards.

professional practice model. The driving force of nursing care; a schematic description of a theory, phenomenon, or system that depicts how nurses practice, collaborate, communicate, and develop professionally to provide the highest quality care for those served by the organization (e.g., patients, families, community). Professional practice models illustrate the alignment and integration of nursing practice with the mission, vision, and values that nursing has adapted.

quality improvement (QI). "Systematic, data-guided activities designed to bring about immediate improvement in healthcare delivery in particular settings" (Lynn et al., 2007, p. 667).

registered nurse (RN). A nurse in the United States who holds state board licensure as a registered nurse or any new graduate or foreign nurse graduate who is awaiting state board examination results and is employed by a healthcare organization with responsibilities of an RN. In other countries, this individual will have registered with the appropriate regulatory body.

research. A systematic investigation, including research development, testing, and evaluation, designed to develop or contribute to generalizable knowledge. (U.S. Department of Health and Human Services, n.d., [45 CFR §46.102(d)] [21 CFR §50.3(k)] [21 CFR §312.3]). Research is distinguished from research utilization, the process of synthesizing, disseminating, and using research-generated knowledge to make an impact on, or a change in, the existing practices in society (Burns and Grove, 2005, p. 750).

setting. A stand-alone practice venue within an entity. The term can be used interchangeably with *facility* where appropriate or necessary.

shared leadership/participative decision-making. A model in which nurses are formally organized to make decisions about clinical practice standards, quality improvement, staff and professional development, and research.

staff nurse. A nurse whose primary responsibility is the provision of direct patient care (does not include clinical specialists).

standard. A norm that expresses an agreed-upon level of performance that has been developed to characterize, measure, and provide guidance for achieving excellence in practice.

strategic plan. A plan resulting from a process of "reviewing the mission, environmental surveillance, and previous planning decisions used to establish major goals and nonrecurring resource allocation decisions" (Griffith and White, 2002, p. 683).

structure. The characteristics of the organization and the healthcare system, including leadership, availability of resources, and professional practice models. Donabedian (1980) defined *structure* as the conditions under which care is provided, including material resources, human resources, and organizational characteristics "such as the organization of the medical and nursing staffs, the presence of teaching and research functions, kinds of supervision and performance review, and methods of paying for care" (see 2003, p. 46).

sufficient examples. Provided to indicate that compliance with a source of evidence is not isolated to a single group or area within the organization. While not every unit or clinical area must be represented, there should be evidence that the attribute exists throughout the breadth and depth of the organization.

system. A group of healthcare entities whose nursing is governed by a CNO as identified in this glossary and whether or not separately legally established as a for-profit or non-profit, corporation, association, sole proprietorship, or partnership.

transformational leadership. Leadership that identifies and communicates vision and values and asks for the involvement of the work group to achieve the vision (Burns, 1978, as cited in Dunham-Taylor, 2000).

turnover. Number of employees who resigned, retired, expired, or were terminated divided by the number employed during the same period.

vacancy rate. Calculated as 1 minus FTEs/WTEs employed divided by FTEs/WTEs budgeted times 100.

American Hospital Association. (2007). *Fast facts on US hospitals* [last updated October 23, 2007]. Last accessed April 7, 2000, from http://www.aha.org/aha/resource-center/Statistics-and-Studies/fast-facts.html.

American Nurses Association. (1979). *The study of credentialing in nursing: A new approach* (Vol. I, Report of the Committee). Kansas City, MO: Author.

American Nurses Association. (2000). *Scope and standards of practice for nursing professional development.* Washington, DC: Author.

American Nurses Association. (2001a). *ANA's bill of rights for registered nurses.* Washington, DC: Author.

American Nurses Association. (2001b). *Code of ethics for nurses, with interpretive statements.* Washington, DC: Author.

American Nurses Association. (2004). *Scope and standards for nurse administrators* (2nd ed.). Washington, DC: Author.

American Nurses Association. (2005). *Principles for nurse staffing* (Appendix A). In *Utilization guide for the ANA principles for nurse staffing* (pp. 20–28). Silver Spring, MD: Author.

American Nurses Credentialing Center. (2004). *Magnet Recognition Program: Application Manual 2005.* Silver Spring, MD: Author.

Burns, J. (1978). *Leadership.* New York: Harper & Row.

Burns, N., & Grove, S. K. (2005). *The practice of nursing research: Conduct, critique, and utilization* (5th ed.). St. Louis, MO: Elsevier.

Centers for Medicare and Medicaid Services. (2006, June). *Revised long-term-care facility resident assessment instrument user's manual* (Version 2.0, rev.). Washington, DC: U.S. Department of Health and Human Services, Author.

Corley, M. C., Minick, P., Elswick, R. K., & Jacobs, M. (2005). Nurse moral distress and ethical work environment. *Nursing Ethics, 12*(4), 382–390.

Donabedian, A. (1980). *The definition of quality and approaches to its assessment.* Ann Arbor, MI: Health Administration Press.

Donabedian, A. (2003). *An introduction to quality assurance in health care.* New York: Oxford University Press.

Dunham-Taylor, J. (2000). Nurse executive transformational leadership found in participative organizations. *Journal of Nursing Administration, 30*(5), 241–250.

Farquharson, J.M. (2004). Liability of the nurse manager. In T.D. Aiken (Ed.), *Legal, ethical, and political issues in nursing* (2nd ed.) (pp. 311-336). Philadelphia, PA: F.A. Davis Company.

Greenhalgh, T. (2004). Diffusion of innovations in service organizations: Systematic review and recommendations. *The Milbank Quarterly, 82,* 581–629.

Griffith, J. R., & White, K. R. (2002). *The well-managed healthcare organization* (5th ed.). Chicago: Health Administration Press.

Hinshaw, A.S. (2002). Building magnetism into health organizations. In M.L. McClure & A.S. Hinshaw (Eds.), *Magnet hospitals revisited: Attraction and retention of professional nurses* (pp. 83-102). Washington, DC: American Nurses Association.

Institute of Medicine. (2003). *Health professions education: A bridge to quality.* Washington, DC: National Academy Press.

Lynn, J., Baily, M. A., Bottrell, M., et al. (2007). The ethics of using quality improvement methods in health care. *Annals of Internal Medicine, 146,* 666–673.

MacDonald, C. (2002). Nurse autonomy as relational. *Nursing Ethics, 9,* 194-201.

National Quality Forum. (2004). *National voluntary consensus standards for nursing home care.* Washington, DC: Author.

Needleman, J., Buerhaus, P., Mattke, S., Stewart, M., & Zelevinsky, K. (2002). Nurse-staffing levels and the quality of care in hospitals. *New England Journal of Medicine, 346*(22), 1715–1722.

Polit, D., & Hungler, B. (1995). *Nursing research: Principles and methods.* Philadelphia: Lippincott.

Sackett, D. L., Straus, S. E., Richardson, W. S., Rosenberg, W., & Haynes, R. B. (2000). *Evidence-based medicine: How to practice and teach EBM* (2nd ed.). Edinburgh: Churchill Livingstone.

Schaufeli, W., Salanova, M., González-romá, V., & Bakker, A. (2002). The measurement of engagement and burnout: A two sample confirmatory factor analytic approach. *Journal of Happiness Studies, 3*(1), 71–92.

Scott, J., & Marshall, G. (Eds.). (2005). *A dictionary of sociology.* New York: Oxford University Press.

Tranmer, J. (2005). Autonomy and decision-making in nursing. In L. McGillis Hall (Ed.), *Quality work environments for nurse and patient safety* (pp. 139-162). Sudbury, MA: Jones and Bartlett Publishers.

Urden, L. D., & Monarch, K. (2002). The ANCC Magnet Recognition Program: Converting research findings into action. In M. L. McClure & A. S. Hinshaw (Eds.), *Magnet hospitals revisited: Attraction and retention of professional nurses* (pp. 103–116). Washington, DC: American Nurses Association.

U.S. Department of Health and Human Services. (n.d.). Code of Federal Regulations Title 45 Public Welfare Part 46: Protection of Human Subjects, Title 21 Food and Drugs Part 50: Protection of Human Subjects. Washington, DC: Author.

Wade, G. (1999). Professional nurse autonomy: Concept analysis and application to nursing education. *Journal of Advanced Nursing, 30,* 310–318.

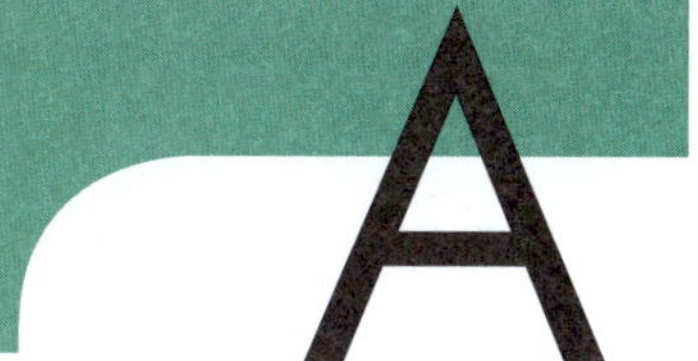

Forces of Magnetism

1. **Quality of nursing leadership**—Nursing leaders were perceived as knowledgeable, strong risk-takers who followed an articulated philosophy in the day-to-day operations of the nursing department. Nursing leaders also conveyed a strong sense of advocacy and support on behalf of the staff.

    Expectations of a Magnet Organization 2005: Knowledgeable, strong, risk-taking nurse leaders follow a well-articulated, strategic, and visionary philosophy in the day-to-day operations of the nursing services. Nursing leaders, at all levels of the organization, convey a strong sense of advocacy and support for the staff and for the patient. (*The results of quality leadership are evident in nursing practice at the patient's side.*)

2. **Organizational structure**—Organizational structures were characterized as flat, rather than tall, and where unit-based decision-making prevailed. Nursing departments were decentralized, with strong nursing representation evident in the organizational committee structure. The nursing leader served at the executive level of the organization, and the chief nursing officer (CNO) reported to the chief executive officer.

    Expectations of a Magnet Organization 2005: Organizational structures are generally flat, rather than tall, and decentralized decision-making prevails. The organizational structure is dynamic and responsive to change. Strong nursing representation is evident in the organizational committee structure. Executive-level nursing leaders serve at the executive level of the organization. The CNO typically reports directly to the chief executive officer. The organization has a functioning and productive system of shared decision-making.

3. **Management style**—Hospital and nursing administrators were found to use a participative management style, incorporating feedback from staff at all levels of the organization. Feedback was characterized as encouraged and valued. Nurses serving in leadership positions were visible, accessible, and committed to communicating effectively with staff.

    Expectations of a Magnet Organization 2005: Healthcare organization and nursing leaders create an environment supporting participation. Feedback is encouraged and valued and is incorporated from the staff at all levels of the organization. Nurses serving in leadership positions are visible, accessible, and committed to communicating effectively with staff.

4. **Personnel policies and programs**—Salaries and benefits were characterized as competitive. Rotating shifts were minimized, and creative and flexible staffing models were used. Personnel polices were created with staff involvement, and significant administrative and clinical promotional opportunities existed.

    Expectations of a Magnet Organization 2005: Salaries and benefits are competitive. Creative and flexible staffing models that support a safe and healthy work environment are used. Personnel policies are created with direct-care nurse involvement. Significant opportunities for professional growth exist in administrative and clinical tracks. Personnel policies and programs support professional nursing practice, work/life balance, and the delivery of quality care.

5. **Professional models of care**—Models of care were used that gave nurses the responsibility and authority for the provision of patient care. Nurses were accountable for their own practice and were the coordinators of care.

   Expectations of a Magnet Organization 2005: There are models of care that give nurses the responsibility and authority for the provision of direct patient care. Nurses are accountable for their own practice as well as the coordination of care. The models of care (i.e., primary nursing, case management, family-centered, district, and holistic) provide for the continuity of care across the continuum. The models take into consideration patients' unique needs and provide skilled nurses and adequate resources to accomplish desired outcomes.

6. **Quality of care**—Nurses perceived that they were providing high-quality care to their patients. Providing quality care was seen as an organizational priority as well, and nurses serving in leadership positions were viewed as responsible for developing the environment in which high-quality care could be provided.

   Expectations of a Magnet Organization 2005: Quality is the systematic driving force for nursing and the organization. Nurses serving in leadership positions are responsible for providing an environment that positively influences patient outcomes. There is a pervasive perception among nurses that they provide high-quality care to patients/residents/clients.

7. **Quality improvement**—Quality improvement activities were viewed as educational. Staff nurses participated in the quality improvement process and perceived the process as one that improved the quality of care delivered within the organization.

   Expectations of a Magnet Organization 2005: The organization has structures and processes for the measurement of quality and programs for improving the quality of care and services within the organization.

8. **Consultation and resources**—Adequate consultation and other human resources were available. Knowledgeable experts, particularly advanced-practice nurses, were available and used. In addition, peer support was given within and outside the nursing division.

   Expectations of a Magnet Organization 2005: The healthcare organization provides adequate resources, support, and opportunities for the utilization of experts, particularly advanced-practice nurses. In addition, the organization promotes involvement of nurses in professional organizations and among peers in the community.

9. **Autonomy**—Nurses were permitted and expected to practice autonomously, consistent with professional standards. Independent judgment was expected to be exercised within the context of a multidisciplinary approach to patient care.

   Expectations of a Magnet Organization 2005: Autonomous nursing care is the ability of a nurse to assess and provide nursing actions as appropriate for patient care based on competence, professional expertise, and knowledge. The nurse is expected to practice autonomously, consistent with professional standards. Independent judgment is expected to be exercised within the context of interdisciplinary and multidisciplinary approaches to patient/resident/client care.

10. **Community and the hospital**—Hospitals that were best able to recruit and retain nurses also maintained a strong community presence. A community presence was seen in a variety of ongoing, long-term outreach programs. These outreach programs resulted in the hospital being perceived as a strong, positive, and productive corporate citizen.

    Expectations of a Magnet Organization 2005: Relationships are established within and among all types of healthcare organizations and other community organizations, to develop strong partnerships that support improved client outcomes and the health of the communities they serve.

11. **Nurses as teachers**—Nurses were permitted and expected to incorporate teaching in all aspects of their practice. Teaching was one activity that reportedly gave nurses a great deal of professional satisfaction.

    Expectations of a Magnet Organization 2005: Professional nurses are involved in educational activities within the organization and community. Students from a variety of academic programs are welcomed and supported in the organization; contractual arrangements are mutually beneficial. There is a development and mentoring program for staff preceptors for all levels of students (e.g., students, new graduates, experienced nurses). Staff in all positions serve as faculty

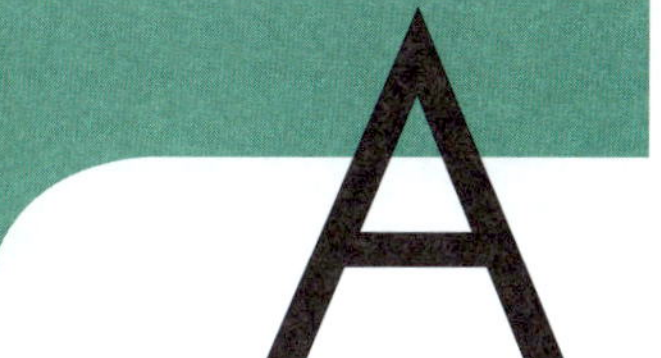

Forces of Magnetism

1. **Quality of nursing leadership**—Nursing leaders were perceived as knowledgeable, strong risk-takers who followed an articulated philosophy in the day-to-day operations of the nursing department. Nursing leaders also conveyed a strong sense of advocacy and support on behalf of the staff.

   Expectations of a Magnet Organization 2005: Knowledgeable, strong, risk-taking nurse leaders follow a well-articulated, strategic, and visionary philosophy in the day-to-day operations of the nursing services. Nursing leaders, at all levels of the organization, convey a strong sense of advocacy and support for the staff and for the patient. (*The results of quality leadership are evident in nursing practice at the patient's side.*)

2. **Organizational structure**—Organizational structures were characterized as flat, rather than tall, and where unit-based decision-making prevailed. Nursing departments were decentralized, with strong nursing representation evident in the organizational committee structure. The nursing leader served at the executive level of the organization, and the chief nursing officer (CNO) reported to the chief executive officer.

   Expectations of a Magnet Organization 2005: Organizational structures are generally flat, rather than tall, and decentralized decision-making prevails. The organizational structure is dynamic and responsive to change. Strong nursing representation is evident in the organizational committee structure. Executive-level nursing leaders serve at the executive level of the organization. The CNO typically reports directly to the chief executive officer. The organization has a functioning and productive system of shared decision-making.

3. **Management style**—Hospital and nursing administrators were found to use a participative management style, incorporating feedback from staff at all levels of the organization. Feedback was characterized as encouraged and valued. Nurses serving in leadership positions were visible, accessible, and committed to communicating effectively with staff.

   Expectations of a Magnet Organization 2005: Healthcare organization and nursing leaders create an environment supporting participation. Feedback is encouraged and valued and is incorporated from the staff at all levels of the organization. Nurses serving in leadership positions are visible, accessible, and committed to communicating effectively with staff.

4. **Personnel policies and programs**—Salaries and benefits were characterized as competitive. Rotating shifts were minimized, and creative and flexible staffing models were used. Personnel polices were created with staff involvement, and significant administrative and clinical promotional opportunities existed.

   Expectations of a Magnet Organization 2005: Salaries and benefits are competitive. Creative and flexible staffing models that support a safe and healthy work environment are used. Personnel policies are created with direct-care nurse involvement. Significant opportunities for professional growth exist in administrative and clinical tracks. Personnel policies and programs support professional nursing practice, work/life balance, and the delivery of quality care.

5. **Professional models of care**—Models of care were used that gave nurses the responsibility and authority for the provision of patient care. Nurses were accountable for their own practice and were the coordinators of care.

   Expectations of a Magnet Organization 2005: There are models of care that give nurses the responsibility and authority for the provision of direct patient care. Nurses are accountable for their own practice as well as the coordination of care. The models of care (i.e., primary nursing, case management, family-centered, district, and holistic) provide for the continuity of care across the continuum. The models take into consideration patients' unique needs and provide skilled nurses and adequate resources to accomplish desired outcomes.

6. **Quality of care**—Nurses perceived that they were providing high-quality care to their patients. Providing quality care was seen as an organizational priority as well, and nurses serving in leadership positions were viewed as responsible for developing the environment in which high-quality care could be provided.

   Expectations of a Magnet Organization 2005: Quality is the systematic driving force for nursing and the organization. Nurses serving in leadership positions are responsible for providing an environment that positively influences patient outcomes. There is a pervasive perception among nurses that they provide high-quality care to patients/residents/clients.

7. **Quality improvement**—Quality improvement activities were viewed as educational. Staff nurses participated in the quality improvement process and perceived the process as one that improved the quality of care delivered within the organization.

   Expectations of a Magnet Organization 2005: The organization has structures and processes for the measurement of quality and programs for improving the quality of care and services within the organization.

8. **Consultation and resources**—Adequate consultation and other human resources were available. Knowledgeable experts, particularly advanced-practice nurses, were available and used. In addition, peer support was given within and outside the nursing division.

   Expectations of a Magnet Organization 2005: The healthcare organization provides adequate resources, support, and opportunities for the utilization of experts, particularly advanced-practice nurses. In addition, the organization promotes involvement of nurses in professional organizations and among peers in the community.

9. **Autonomy**—Nurses were permitted and expected to practice autonomously, consistent with professional standards. Independent judgment was expected to be exercised within the context of a multidisciplinary approach to patient care.

   Expectations of a Magnet Organization 2005: Autonomous nursing care is the ability of a nurse to assess and provide nursing actions as appropriate for patient care based on competence, professional expertise, and knowledge. The nurse is expected to practice autonomously, consistent with professional standards. Independent judgment is expected to be exercised within the context of interdisciplinary and multidisciplinary approaches to patient/resident/client care.

10. **Community and the hospital**—Hospitals that were best able to recruit and retain nurses also maintained a strong community presence. A community presence was seen in a variety of ongoing, long-term outreach programs. These outreach programs resulted in the hospital being perceived as a strong, positive, and productive corporate citizen.

    Expectations of a Magnet Organization 2005: Relationships are established within and among all types of healthcare organizations and other community organizations, to develop strong partnerships that support improved client outcomes and the health of the communities they serve.

11. **Nurses as teachers**—Nurses were permitted and expected to incorporate teaching in all aspects of their practice. Teaching was one activity that reportedly gave nurses a great deal of professional satisfaction.

    Expectations of a Magnet Organization 2005: Professional nurses are involved in educational activities within the organization and community. Students from a variety of academic programs are welcomed and supported in the organization; contractual arrangements are mutually beneficial. There is a development and mentoring program for staff preceptors for all levels of students (e.g., students, new graduates, experienced nurses). Staff in all positions serve as faculty and preceptors for students from a variety of academic programs. There is a patient education program that meets the diverse needs of patients in all of the care settings of the organization.

12. **Image of nursing**—Nurses were viewed as integral to the hospital's ability to provide patient care services. The services provided by nurses were characterized as essential to other members of the healthcare team.

    Expectations of a Magnet Organization 2005: The services provided by nurses are characterized as essential by other members of the healthcare team. Nurses are viewed as integral to the healthcare organization's ability to provide patient care. Nurses effectively influence system-wide processes.

13. **Interdisciplinary relationships**—Interdisciplinary relationships were characterized as positive. A sense of mutual respect was exhibited among all disciplines.

    Expectations of a Magnet Organization 2005: Collaborative working relationships within and among the disciplines are valued. Mutual respect is based on the premise that all members of the healthcare team make essential and meaningful contributions in the achievement of clinical outcomes. Conflict management strategies are in place and are used effectively, when indicated.

14. **Professional development**—Significant emphasis was placed on orientation, in-service education, continuing education, formal education, and career development. Personal and professional growth and development were valued. In addition, opportunities for competency-based clinical advancement existed, along with the resources to maintain competency.

    Expectations of a Magnet Organization 2005: The healthcare organization values and supports the personal and professional growth and development of staff. In addition to quality orientation and in-service education addressed earlier in Force 11, emphasis is placed on providing career development services. Programs that promote formal education, professional certification, and career development are evident. Competency-based clinical and leadership/management development is promoted, and adequate human and fiscal resources for all professional development programs are provided.

Sources: American Nurses Credentialing Center (2004, pp. 36–65), Urden and Monarch (2002, pp. 106–107).

APPENDIX B
Crosswalk from 2005 to 2008

KEY:

TL	Transformational Leadership	SE	Structural Empowerment
EP	Exemplary Professional Performance	NK	New Knowledge
EO	Empirical Outcomes	OO	Organizational Overview

	2005 *MANUAL* SOURCE OF EVIDENCE	2008 LOCATION
OO1	Information describing the applicant organization in terms of geographical location, services provided, number of beds, number of employees, and population served. Include the most recent demographic report regarding the client population that the organization is serving.	OO1
OO2	An administrative organizational chart and a nursing organizational chart.	OO5
OO3	Provide a list and explanatory documentation of any unfair labor practice charges involving a nurse (whether pending, arbitrated, or dismissed) that have been brought against the applicant organization before the NLRB, state, or international court within the 3-year period prior to the submission of this application.	deleted
OO4	State Nurse Practice Act. It is sufficient to provide the web address of this document after validating that the most current version of the state Nurse Practice Act is available on the web site. If this is not the case, provide a hard copy of the most current version of the state Nurse Practice Act.	OO16
OO5	For U.S. applicants, case mix index information, by service/product line, for each of the two (2) 1-year periods immediately preceding the submission of written documentation.	OO14
OO6	Total Nursing Care Hours/Patient Day (HPPD) by unit for each of the two (2) 1-year periods immediately preceding the submission of written documentation.	OO11
OO7	A description, signed by the chief executive officer (CEO), summarizing, from the CEO perspective, the investment and commitment the organization has made to recruiting and retaining nurses, resource allocation for excellence-focused management of patients/residents/ clients so that desired client-centered outcomes are achieved, the relationship and consistency between the goals and priorities of nursing and those of the organization, as well as the accomplishments, advances, contributions, and innovations realized within nursing.	deleted

		2005 *MANUAL* SOURCE OF EVIDENCE	2008 LOCATION
	OO8	A description, signed by the chief financial officer (CFO), summarizing, from the CFO perspective, the investment and commitment the organization has made to recruiting and retaining nurses, resource allocation for excellence-focused management of patients/residents/clients so that desired client-centered outcomes are achieved, the relationship and consistency between the goals and priorities of nursing and those of the organization, as well as the accomplishments, advances, contributions, and innovations realized within nursing.	deleted
	OO9	A description of the issues with which the organization has zero tolerance, including, but not limited to, harassment of any type, workplace violence, and discrimination.	deleted
	OO10a	CNO job description.	OO2
	OO10b	CNO performance appraisals for each year for the 2 years immediately preceding the submission of written documentation (if the CNO has been in place for less than 2 years, then one (1) performance appraisal will be acceptable).	deleted
	OO10c	Evidence that the CNO has been in place for at least 1 year prior to the submission of written documentation.	deleted
	OO10d	Evidence that the CNO, or his or her designee, participates in the privileging process for advanced-practice nurses.	OO18
	OO10e	Description of the CNO's mentoring activities that have been engaged in, as well as activities that have been completed to promote the profession of nursing, including, but not limited to, public speaking and submitting articles for publication in the nursing literature.	TL6
	OO10f	A list and/or description of the CNO's professional development activities that have been engaged in during the 2-year period immediately preceding the submission of written documentation.	OO6
	OO11	Any information related to any violations of any regulations or laws that have been substantiated against the organization within the past 5-year period immediately preceding the submission of written documentation.	deleted
	OO12	The organization's and the nursing division's most recent annual report.	OO3
	OO13	Mission, vision, strategic plan, and priorities, as well as the performance improvement plan of both the organization and the nursing division.	OO1
	OO14	Theoretical/practice framework(s) stylized within the nursing division that structures various aspects of professional practice (e.g., patient care, nursing research, staff development, performance evaluation and improvement) and performance.	OO11, EP1
	OO15	Methods that are used to meet patient needs. A description of the mechanism(s) used to ensure that an appropriate skill mix of adequate numbers of staff are available.	EP8
	OO16	The satisfaction survey completed by nurses who provide direct patient/client/resident care in the past 12-month period.	OO13, EP3, EP3EO
	OO17	Organizational policies and procedures related to confidentiality of patient personal information, the documentation of patients'/residents'/clients' care activities, and staffing. Organizational policies and procedures related to confidentiality of staff personal information.	deleted
	OO18	A description of the steps taken and mechanisms put in place to ensure that patients/residents/clients are cared for in a safe and healthful environment.	OO21, EP31, EP32, EP32EO
	OO19	A description of the steps taken and mechanisms put in place to ensure that nurses practice in a safe and healthful environment.	EP30, EP30EO, EP31

	2005 *MANUAL* SOURCE OF EVIDENCE	2008 LOCATION
OO20	Identification of important/key changes made in the nursing division as a result of data gained from participating in national, benchmarkable studies regarding quality, productivity, safety, and costs associated with delivering services to clients.	deleted
OO21	A description of the steps taken within the organization to address the identified needs of nurse employees.	TL10, deleted

	2005 *MANUAL* SOURCE OF EVIDENCE	2008 LOCATION
1.1	Describe how the mission, vision, values, philosophy, and strategic plan of nursing services are congruent with those aspects of the organization.	TL1
1.2	Describe how the CNO includes nurses who work in areas other than nursing services in activities and decision-making regarding nursing care.	OO5, TL10
1.3	Give examples, from several different nursing units, of advocacy by the CNO on behalf of the staff, such as requests for additional FTEs, systems, equipment, personnel support, and so forth.	TL2
1.4	Provide examples of how nurses at all levels are leading and participating in professional nursing organizations and activities at the local, state, national, and/or international levels. Include examples of how this benefits the practice setting and the nursing community.	SE11EO, SE2, SE2EO
1.5	Describe the involvement of nurses at all levels in the budget development process.	OO4, EP12
1.6	Provide evidence of data-driven decision-making regarding budget formulation, implementation, monitoring, and evaluation.	OO4, EP12
1.7	Provide specific examples of ways nurses at all levels have identified and advocated for additional nursing resources to support unit goals.	TL2
1.8	Provide nurse satisfaction data for a 2-year period. Describe how nurse-satisfaction data are tracked and analyzed and how action plans are developed and evaluated based on data. Address how direct-care nurses are involved in the process.	OO13, EP3, EP3EO

	2005 *MANUAL* SOURCE OF EVIDENCE	2008 LOCATION
2.1	Provide a narrative and supportive evidence from nursing and non-nursing executive leadership that describes the CNO's structural and operational relationships with organizational leaders.	deleted
2.2	Provide evidence of the CNO's position and influence on the organization's highest decision-making body.	OO5, TL4
2.3	Provide a narrative that describes the CNO's structural and operational relationships in all areas where nursing is practiced.	OO5
2.4	Describe how the CNO has enabled decentralized decision-making through education, facilitation, and support.	OO10, SE, SE1EO
2.5	Describe how decision-making is operationalized to involve all levels of nurses.	TL2
2.6	Provide examples of how the organizational structure has been modified to accommodate change from an internal or external force.	TL10, TL10EO

		2005 *MANUAL* SOURCE OF EVIDENCE	2008 LOCATION
3.1		Describe the CNO's leadership style and give at least two (2) examples related to the components referenced above.	TL8
3.2		Provide examples of effective and ineffective leadership-style outcomes and follow-up action as appropriate.	TL5
3.3		Provide examples of how direct-care nurses' feedback is used in organizational decision-making.	SE1, SE1EO, TL2, TL10
3.4		Describe mechanisms or processes that create a practice environment that fosters horizontal and vertical communication between nurses at all levels throughout the organization.	TL8, TL9
3.5		Provide examples of how direct-care nurses initiate change to improve patient care, nursing practice, and/or the work environment.	TL10, EP22
3.6		Provide examples of how direct-care nurses' feedback is used by nurse leaders to make changes to improve patient care, nursing practice, and/or the work environment.	TL10, TL10EO
3.7		4. Describe how nursing leaders are visible and accessible to direct-care nurses.	TL8, TL9
3.8		6. Provide examples of mentoring and succession planning by and for nurse leaders and direct-care nurses.	TL6

		2005 *MANUAL* SOURCE OF EVIDENCE	2008 LOCATION
4.1		Describe the formal and informal performance appraisal processes used in the organization, including self-appraisal, peer review, and 360o evaluation (as appropriate) for nurses at all levels in the organization.	OO17, EP20
4.2		Provide examples of how workplace advocacy policies and procedures safeguard employee rights and promote a safe and healthy work environment.	OO20, OO21, OO22, EP29
4.3		Describe how staffing plans and practices are consistent with the *ANA Principles for Nurse Staffing*.	EP11
4.4		Describe how the organization fosters a nondiscriminatory climate in which care is delivered in a manner that is sensitive to diversity.	EP25, EP27
4.5		Provide examples of how the organization addresses workforce diversity.	EP27
4.6		Describe the organization's nursing recruitment and retention programs and responses to ongoing challenges in the marketplace.	EP10
4.7		Provide action plans developed with direct-care nurse input/involvement to address variation in unit- or service-based turnover and vacancy rates.	EP10
4.8		Provide examples of how direct-care nurses participate in recruitment and retention activities.	EP10
4.9		Illustrate the ongoing collaborative efforts of nursing, finance, and human resources related to personnel policies and programs.	SE3, SE4, SE5, SE6, SE7
4.10		Demonstrate how trending data are used in the formulation of the staffing plan and to acquire necessary resources.	EP8, EP9
4.11		Provide representative examples of the development of unit staffing plans and corresponding schedules.	deleted
4.12		Explain how staffing adjustments are made in response to fluctuating patient workload and acuity (e.g., use of agency, float staff, overtime).	EP8
4.13		Describe alterations in scheduling practices related to budget variance analyses.	deleted

	2005 *MANUAL* SOURCE OF EVIDENCE	2008 LOCATION
4.14	Relate the delegation activities of direct-care nurses to the requirements of the state Nurse Practice Act, other regulatory stipulations, and professional standards.	EP11
4.15	Demonstrate mechanisms by which direct-care nurses are educated about matching staff assignments to patient needs and staff member skill sets and experience.	OO10
4.16	Provide representative examples of patient assignments, including the rationale for the assignments of personnel of various roles, who was responsible for making assignments, and who had input into the process.	EP5
4.17	Provide examples that the organization supports career development opportunities for organization employees interested in becoming nurses or nurse support staff.	SE6
4.18	Provide examples of how the performance appraisal processes improve the practice of nurses at the direct-care and the nurse administrator levels.	EP20

	2005 *MANUAL* SOURCE OF EVIDENCE	2008 LOCATION
5.1	Detail how the state Nurse Practice Act, other regulatory stipulations (e.g., staffing ratios recently mandated in California), and professional standards influence the care delivery model(s).	OO10, EP6
5.2	Detail how the state Nurse Practice Act, other regulatory stipulations, and professional standards are incorporated into the development, implementation, and evaluation of professional models of care.	EP6
5.3	Describe how direct-care nurses are educated regarding the tenets of the state Nurse Practice Act, other regulatory documents, and professional standards.	OO10
5.4	Demonstrate how the state Nurse Practice Act, other regulatory stipulations, and professional standards are available as references on each unit and incorporated into daily decisions.	EP19
5.5	Describe the role of the direct-care nurse in the development, implementation, and evaluation of care delivery models.	EP1
5.6	Describe how the model of care addresses patient needs, patient population demographics, number of nursing staff members, and ratio of nurses serving in various roles and levels.	deleted
5.7	Describe innovations by direct-care nurses to implement the model of care and to meet the needs of specific patient populations at the unit level.	EP25, EP26
5.8	Describe how the continuity of the patient's care is addressed in the professional model(s) for the delivery of patient care.	EP5
5.9	Provide representative examples that depict the scheduling process, and describe how scheduling is tailored to the patient population, unit needs, and the needs of individual staff members.	EP8, EP9
5.10	Provide several examples of how direct-care nurses influence scheduling.	EP9
5.11	Describe how the various levels of nurse leaders ensure that the utilization of personnel resources is consistent with the established staffing plan, scheduling plan, patient needs, and model of care.	EP5, EP8

		2005 *MANUAL* SOURCE OF EVIDENCE	2008 LOCATION
	6.1	Describe the quality infrastructure—the organizational committees and decision-making bodies that affect client care—and the involvement of nurses from various settings and at all levels of the organization in establishing, monitoring, and evaluating practice standards and patient care policies at the unit and organizational levels.	OO10, OO25, EP2, EP33
	6.2	Provide evidence that direct-care nurses perceive they are providing high-quality patient care.	deleted
	6.3	Give an example to illustrate how the allocation of human and material resources has improved the quality of patient care.	EP33EO
	6.4	Describe the processes by which standards of practice and standards of care are developed, implemented, monitored for impact, and systematically evaluated at the organizational and unit levels.	OO10, EP2, NK6, NK7, NK7EO
	6.5	Describe how each step of the nursing process is operationalized in nursing practice throughout the organization.	deleted
	6.6	Describe the process by which innovative patient safety programs or initiatives have been developed, implemented, and evaluated. Include examples that demonstrate the involvement of nurses from various practice settings and at all levels, and that demonstrate how these programs or initiatives have improved patient safety outcomes.	OO23, TL7, EP32, EP32EO
	6.7	Describe the process by which staff safety programs have been developed, implemented, and evaluated.	OO24, EP30, EP30EO
	6.8	Provide policies and procedures that address the identification and management of problems related to incompetent, unsafe, or unethical practice. Give examples to illustrate compliance with these policies.	OO20, OO21, EP28
	6.9	Provide evidence that nurses have access to avenues for confidential and anonymous reporting of unsafe practice or unsafe environmental factors without recrimination.	OO20, EP28
	6.10	Describe organizational support, resources, and initiatives that have improved workplace safety for nurses.	OO24, EP30, EP30EO, EP31
	6.11	Describe policies and procedures for ensuring protection of confidentiality, privacy, and security for patients and staff and monitoring systems for ensuring compliance.	OO10, EP24
	6.12	Describe how the ANA *Code of Ethics for Nurses* is adhered to across the nursing organization.	EP23
	6.13	Describe processes for educating patients and families about the Patient's Bill of Rights, processes for the dissemination of the Patient's Bill of Rights, and examples to illustrate how the Patient's Bill of Rights shapes organizational policy and practice.	deleted
	6.14	Describe how the nurses are educated about the Bill of Rights for Registered Nurses and how it is implemented across the organization.	OO10, EP23
	6.15	Provide examples that show how nurses at all levels are educated in applying ethical principles in nursing practice.	OO10
	6.16	Provide examples that show how nurses are supported in applying ethical principles in nursing practice.	OO19, EP23, EP24
	6.17	Give examples of programs, services, and initiatives developed to meet the cultural, ethical, and demographic needs of a diverse patient population and the resources, fiscal and human, allocated to support these programs, services, and initiatives.	EP25, EP26
	6.18	Provide data that compare and contrast the ethnicity of the organization's service area, with the ethnicity of inpatients/residents for the most recent fiscal year, and include an ethnic profile of the professional nursing staff.	OO1

	2005 *MANUAL* SOURCE OF EVIDENCE	2008 LOCATION
6.19	Describe how the nursing organization prepares the professional staff to meet the projected needs of diverse populations.	OO10
6.20	Provide copies of structure and process standards (policies and procedures) that reflect how the organization addresses patient/resident language and hearing needs.	EP26
6.21	Provide evidence of workplace advocacy efforts that have improved the work environment for nurses at all levels.	EP29, EP30, EP30EO
6.22	Describe how current literature, appropriate to the practice setting, is available, disseminated, and used to change administrative and clinical practices.	EP19, NK1
6.23	Discuss the institution's policies and procedures that protect the rights of participants in research protocols. Include evidence of consistent nursing involvement in the governing body responsible for protection of human subjects in research.	OO27, NK2, NK3
6.24	Provide evidence that research consultants are actively involved in shaping nursing research infrastructure, capacity, and mentorship.	OO28
6.25	Provide a copy of the nursing budget or other sources of funding for the past year, the current year-to-date, and the future projection, highlighting the allocation and utilization of resources for nursing research.	OO4, NK4
6.26	Supply documentation of all nursing research activities that are ongoing, including internal validation studies, internal and external research, and participation in surveys completed within the past 12-month period.	NK4EO
6.27	Provide evidence of education and mentoring activities that have effectively engaged staff nurses in research and/or evidence-based practice activities.	OO10, NK3
6.28	Describe resources available to nursing staff to support participation in nursing research and nursing research utilization activities.	OO4, NK4, NK6, NK7

	2005 *MANUAL* SOURCE OF EVIDENCE	2008 LOCATION
7.1	Describe the organization's quality plan and the relationship of nursing quality initiatives at the departmental and unit level to the plan.	OO3, TL1
7.2	Describe the role and accountability of the CNO related to quality improvement. Give an example to demonstrate how the CNO has effectively influenced system-level change to improve the quality of care.	TL4, TL4EO
7.3	Explain the mechanisms for ensuring comprehensive dissemination of quality data to all stakeholders in the organization and illustrate the process with a representative example.	EP34
7.4	Describe the processes and rationale for the identification, development, and utilization of national databases that include nursing-sensitive measures that impact client-centered outcomes.	OO23, EP32, EP32EO
7.5	Provide an example at the organizational, departmental, or unit level of a change in practice that resulted from an integrated analysis of data from fiscal, human resource, clinical outcomes, and/or satisfaction survey sources.	OO23, OO26, EP3, EP3EO, EP33, EP33EO, EP35, EP35EO
7.6	For clinical areas that are not included in national databases, explain how benchmarks and nursing-sensitive measures are selected, implemented, and evaluated by nurses at the organizational, departmental, and unit levels to improve patient outcomes.	deleted
7.7	Give examples to demonstrate how the nursing department communicates expectations of direct-care nurses' accountability for quality improvement activities.	OO10

	2005 *MANUAL* SOURCE OF EVIDENCE	2008 LOCATION
7.8	Give examples to demonstrate how the nursing department provides the resources, education, and support to facilitate staff involvement in quality improvement activities.	OO10, EP33, EP34
7.9	Provide examples of nurse involvement in evidence-based quality initiatives to improve coordination and delivery of care across the continuum of services.	EP5, NK7EO

	2005 *MANUAL* SOURCE OF EVIDENCE	2008 LOCATION
8.1	Describe how leadership establishes a practice environment in which resources—from within the organization as well as from sources external to the organization—are developed and/or procured to support professional nursing practice for nurses at all levels in the organization.	EP7
8.2	Describe the processes that ensure that adequate resources for consultation and access to nursing experts (expertise) are available to nurses at all levels in the organization.	deleted
8.3	Describe the organization's relationships with educational institutions (including schools of nursing) for consultation and building a collaborative/professional nursing community.	SE11
8.4	Describe how leadership facilitates and supports participation of nurses at all levels in the organization in professional nursing organizations.	OO7, SE2
8.5	Describe how leadership facilitates and supports participation of nurses at all levels in the organization in healthcare and community organizations other than professional nursing organizations.	SE11
8.6	Describe how the organization utilizes advanced-practice nurses.	EP7
8.7	Give examples of how networking activities, professional organization participation, and use of consultants and advanced-practice nurses have contributed to enhancing patient outcomes.	SE2EO, EP7EO
8.8	Give examples of how networking activities, professional organization participation, and use of consultants and advanced-practice nurses have contributed to enhancing the practice of nurses at all levels in the organization through enhancement of their knowledge and skills.	EP7EO

	2005 *MANUAL* SOURCE OF EVIDENCE	2008 LOCATION
9.1	Describe the process by which advanced practice nurses are credentialed, privileged, and evaluated.	OO17
9.2	Describe how the organization ensures that nurses in all settings practice autonomously and in accordance with national professional nursing standards.	SE1, EP2, EP14, EP19, EP21
9.3	Demonstrate how direct-care nurses use available professional standards, literature, and research findings to support control over nursing practice, independent decision-making, and assertiveness/leadership in patient care management and practice. Provide evidence from multiple patient care settings within the organization.	EP2, EP19, NK1, NK7
9.4	Provide examples of issues that were identified by direct-care nurses, and that affected patient outcomes, and how said issues were addressed.	TL10, TL10EO, EP24
9.5	Describe how opportunities for independent, intra-dependent, and interdependent nursing practice for direct-care nurses are developed and initiated, including required educational programs and continuing competence evaluations.	deleted

	2005 *MANUAL* SOURCE OF EVIDENCE	2008 LOCATION
9.6	Provide evidence that nurses throughout the organization have access to the Internet, library, and/or other appropriate literature/data sources.	EP19, NK1
9.7	Describe how the peer review process is used for professional growth for nurses at all levels in the organization.	EP20
9.8	Describe examples in which staff nurses exercise independent judgment to resolve patient care issues.	EP22, EP24

	2005 *MANUAL* SOURCE OF EVIDENCE	2008 LOCATION
10.1	Describe partnerships established by the organization and/or by nurse leaders with community-based entities to advance nursing practice within the organization.	SE11
10.2	Describe partnerships and programs established by the nursing department with community-based entities to meet the healthcare needs of the populations served.	SE13
10.3	Describe nurse involvement in the community (meant to be personal, such as Red Cross volunteers, Habitat for Humanity, school presentations, etc.).	SE12
10.4	Discuss the process for fiscal allocations for nursing affiliations (e.g., nursing schools, nurse researchers, consortium work, outreach programs).	SE11
10.5	Explain how the organization supports/encourages nurse involvement in the community. Specifically, explain how nurses are compensated (as appropriate) for this community effort.	SE12
10.6	Discuss expectations for participation in community activities found in position descriptions and performance evaluations.	deleted
10.7	Provide examples of outcomes resulting from community collaborations/ partnerships, including clinical and fiscal elements, and evidence of overall community impact.	SE11EO
10.8	Describe programs and outcomes that have resulted from nursing collaborations/partnerships with other nursing entities in the community (e.g., nursing schools, nurse researchers, consortium work, outreach programs) or region.	SE11, SE11EO
10.9	Describe awards/recognitions received by the facility or its employees for community support/involvement.	SE15

	2005 *MANUAL* SOURCE OF EVIDENCE	2008 LOCATION
11.1	Describe the process of assessing, planning, organizing, implementing, and evaluating the educational needs of nurses at all levels of the organization.	OO9, SE5, SE5EO
11.2	Describe how the transition of new graduate nurses is facilitated.	SE8
11.3	Describe the orientation and continuing education developed for clinicians, administrators, and other nursing-role specialties at all levels of the organization.	OO9, SE5, SE5EO
11.4	Describe and provide evidence of mentoring activities at all levels of the organization for both clinical and leadership roles.	TL6
11.5	Give examples of organizational incentives (e.g., clinical ladder promotion criteria, position descriptions, standardized care plans, clinical pathways) that promote the nurse teaching role.	SE7
11.6	Delineate staff involvement as faculty/adjunct faculty.	SE10

		2005 *MANUAL* SOURCE OF EVIDENCE	2008 LOCATION
11.7		Describe all innovative, creative academic practicum experiences that are in place in the organization.	SE10
11.8		Describe the process of assessing, planning, organizing, implementing, and evaluating the educational needs, reflecting concern for cultural differences and language, of patient populations at all levels of the organization.	SE7, EP25, EP26
11.9		Provide examples of specialty- or population-based patient education initiatives conducted, implemented, and evaluated by nurses.	SE7
11.10		Give examples of community collaborative educational endeavors (e.g., guest lectures for affiliating agencies).	SE9
11.11		Provide evidence of broad participation in professional development programs designed to develop, refine, and enhance teaching of expertise.	SE9

		2005 *MANUAL* SOURCE OF EVIDENCE	2008 LOCATION
12.1		Provide examples to illustrate how the CNO has influenced organizational decision-making and strategic planning.	TL4, TL4EO
12.2		Provide evidence that the CNO is viewed by organization stakeholders as having equal status with other senior decision-makers.	TL4
12.3		Provide evidence of how the organization recognizes the contribution of nurses toward the achievement of strategic priorities and makes these contributions visible within the organization.	SE14
12.4		Provide examples of the good relationship(s) between nursing and other departments.	EP15, EP16, EP17, EP18
12.5		Give examples of how nurses in nontraditional roles (e.g., informatics, group facilitation, organizational performance, staff development, resource analysis) have had a positive impact on the image of nursing within the organization.	deleted
12.6		Provide examples of how nursing is featured in the organization's promotional advertising strategies and materials, including newsletters, bulletin boards, Internet sites, published leadership profiles, and so forth.	deleted
12.7		Give examples of how interdisciplinary teams perceive nursing in the organization.	deleted
12.8		Give examples of how the community perceives nursing as well as nursing services provided within the organization.	SE15

		2005 *MANUAL* SOURCE OF EVIDENCE	2008 LOCATION
13.1		Describe mechanisms used to ensure and/or promote the participation of the nurses at all levels in interdisciplinary activities.	EP13
13.2		Submit a list of all committees and/or task forces and their nurse membership, roles, and work locations within the organization.	OO15
13.3		Provide the policy or operating guidelines for committees and/or task forces within the organization that include representatives of nursing, detailing committee membership requirements and voting privileges.	OO15
13.4		Provide three examples of interdisciplinary collaboration in which nurses have assumed a leadership role.	EP12, EP13
13.5		Describe the formal mechanisms that govern organizational operations at the senior policy-making level, including membership, voting privileges, and/or processes typically used in decision-making activities.	deleted

		2005 *MANUAL* SOURCE OF EVIDENCE	2008 LOCATION
	13.6	Provide examples of documentation systems/tools used in patient care planning and interdisciplinary communication during the 12 months prior to application submission.	EP17
	13.7	Provide at least two (2) patient/resident exemplars/case studies that demonstrate interdisciplinary collaboration across multiple settings, such as acute care, extended care facilities, and home care, highlighting the cooperation and collaboration between and among healthcare team members.	EP16
	13.8	Provide at least one (1) example of interdisciplinary involvement in addressing patient-centered clinical outcomes.	EP15
	13.9	Provide at least one (1) example of interdisciplinary involvement in addressing policy development.	EP13, EP14
	13.10	Provide at least one (1) example of interdisciplinary involvement in addressing nursing governance.	deleted
	13.11	Provide at least one (1) example of interdisciplinary involvement in addressing establishing inter/intradepartmental standards.	EP13, EP14
	13.12	Provide at least one (1) example of interdisciplinary involvement in addressing decision-making related to the allocation of scarce resources.	EP18
	13.13	Provide at least one (1) example of interdisciplinary involvement in addressing continuous quality/process improvement.	EP15
	13.14	Provide at least one (1) example of interdisciplinary involvement in addressing fiscal planning.	deleted
	13.15	Provide at least one (1) example of interdisciplinary involvement in addressing the facility's development or remodeling projects.	deleted
	13.16	Describe the process by which all levels of nurses participate in the evaluation of nursing standards and detail mechanisms for the inclusion of other disciplines, where indicated.	EP2, EP13
	13.17	Describe the approach that governs the management of interdisciplinary conflict, including a description of the most recent use of this approach and resulting outcomes thereof.	OO22

		2005 *MANUAL* SOURCE OF EVIDENCE	2008 LOCATION
	14.1	Describe professional development programs, such as tuition reimbursement; access to web-based education; and participation in local, regional, national, and international conferences/meetings. Supply the structure and process standards (policies and procedures) that govern/guide these programs.	OO8, SE4
	14.2	Submit a report that details the continuing education activities, self-directed learning activities, and attendance at nursing and interdisciplinary conferences of the CNO and nurse executive leadership group for the 12 months prior to the application submission.	OO6
	14.3	Submit a report that details the formal educational activities of the CNO and the nurse executive leadership group for the 12 months prior to application submission.	OO6
	14.4	Submit a report that details how education is provided regarding ethical issues, nursing research, and evidence-based practice, and include learning objectives, a content outline, and numbers of employees (specifically identifying the number of nurses) who were educated in the 12 months prior to application submission.	OO10

MAGNET DICTIONARY

acute care
A healthcare organization in which care is delivered to hospitalized patients.

		2005 *MANUAL* SOURCE OF EVIDENCE	2008 LOCATION
14.5		Describe how the healthcare organization provides employee education regarding patient/resident privacy, security, and confidentiality rights. Detail the frequency of such offerings; provide presentation objectives, a content outline, and numbers of employees (specifically identifying the number of nurses) who were educated in the 12 months prior to application submission.	OO10
14.6		Submit a report that details, on a clinical unit basis, the financial support expended to support nurses attending educational programs or conferences outside the healthcare organization.	OO4
14.7		Describe how the development of cultural competence in the professional healthcare staff is promoted and supported.	OO10, EP25, EP27
14.8		Describe the participation/involvement of nurses at all levels in the activities of professional organizations.	SE2
14.9		Submit a report that details, on a clinical unit basis, the participation of the direct-care nurses in continuing education programs during the 12 months prior to application submission. List the number of continuing education offerings and the percentage of nurses (on a unit basis) who attended each offering.	deleted
14.10		Identify clinical skills and/or competencies recognized by nursing as requiring formal credentialing and privileging mechanisms.	deleted
14.11		Describe how nurse administrators ensure that direct-care nurses achieve clinical competency and leadership skills.	TL6, SE4, SE4EO, SE5
14.12		Describe how professional certification across all nursing roles (administration and clinical practice) is promoted by the healthcare organization.	SE4
14.13		Describe the structure and process standards that govern/guide the privileging and credentialing of professional nurses to perform specific clinical skills or competencies recognized by nursing as requiring formal credentialing and privileging mechanisms.	deleted
14.14		Submit a report that details leadership development programs that have been offered on topics such as delegation, the change process, and conflict management during the 12 months prior to application submission.	OO10, TL6
14.15		Provide a report that details the academic credentials of the nurse administrators, formal academic programs in which currently enrolled and earned professional certification.	OO6

2008 Manual New Sources of Evidence	2008 Location
New	OO9
New	OO20
New	TL3
New	TL3EO
New	TL7
New	SE3
New	EP4
New	EP24
New	NK5
New	NK8
New	NK9
New	NK9EO

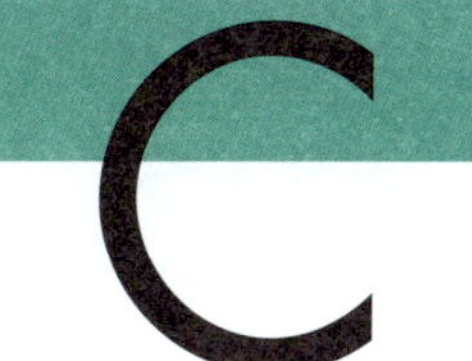

Long-Term-Care and Home Care Nursing Sensitive Indicators

INDICATORS FOR LONG-TERM-CARE ORGANIZATIONS/UNITS

MAGNET DICTIONARY

long-term care
A healthcare organization in which elderly and frail individuals reside.

Long-term-care applicants must collect, analyze, and report data benchmarked at the highest available level. In addition, long-term-care applicants must collect and report on those indicators currently sponsored by the Center for Medicare & Medicaid Services (CMS) through the Minimum Data Set (MDS). Long-term-care applicants also may select indicators for nursing home care developed by the National Quality Forum (NQF, 2004). If the long-term-care applicant selects NQF indicators, they may be used in lieu of the CMS indicators, *only* for the same category.

INDICATORS FOR HOME CARE ORGANIZATIONS/UNITS

Home care applicants must collect, analyze, and report data benchmarked at the highest available level. In addition, home care applicants must collect and report on those indicators currently sponsored by the CMS through the Outcome and Assessment Information Set (OASIS; Centers for Medicare and Medicaid Services, 2006; http://www.cms.hhs.gov/NursingHomeQualityInits/20_NHQIMDS20.asp).

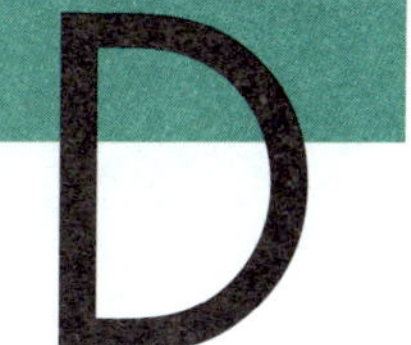

Application as a System

SYSTEM ELIGIBILITY REQUIREMENTS

Each entity within a system must demonstrate the development, dissemination, and enculturation of each Force of Magnetism. Applicants applying as a system must meet each of the following requirements in addition to the requirements listed in Chapter 2. Applicant organizations with component entities in different states will be addressed on a case-by-case basis.

Transformational Leadership
- There must be one organizational mission, vision, and set of values for the entire system.
- There must be one chief executive officer for the entire system.
- There must be one governing board for the entire system.
- The same shared leadership/participative decision-making mechanism must be operationalized throughout the entire system.
- There must be one chief nursing officer (CNO) for the entire system.
- Each component entity shall have a designated RN executive leader who:
    - Is prominently responsible for nursing service at that entity;
    - Has detailed knowledge and control over the day-to-day operations of the clinical practice of nursing within that entity; and
    - Meets the CNO educational requirements.
- There must be an established nursing council/committee in which representatives from all component entities participate in shared decision-making and developing strategy for system-wide nursing initiatives.
- The component entities must demonstrate how nurses participate in shared decision-making.

Structural Empowerment
- The same educational opportunities, to include orientation, certification, clinical ladders, and financial support in budget, must exist across the entire system.
- There must be an integrated nursing education department serving the entire system.
- There must be an established system-wide patient and family education committee.
- The same support for nursing research, to include personnel and finance, must exist throughout the entire system.
- There must be system-wide nursing participation in a community advisory committee.

- There must be system-wide nursing participation in community-sponsored events.
- There must be system-wide marketing and integration of publications that are promoted to the community and nursing staff.

Exemplary Professional Practice

- The same mission, vision, and values must be used throughout the system.
- The same performance appraisals must be used throughout the system.
- The same pay practices must be used throughout the system.
- The same policies and procedures must be used throughout the system.
- The same policies supporting career development and advancement must be used throughout the system.
- The same credentialing and privileging process for advanced-practice nurses must exist throughout the entire system.
- The same clinical documentation system(s) must be used throughout the system to support integration of evidence-based practice into clinical and operational processes.
- The same policies and procedures governing interdisciplinary relationships must be applied across the entire system.
- The same performance improvement methodology/structure must exist throughout the entire system.

Knowledge Improvement

- The same clinical documentation system(s) must be used throughout the system to support integration of research into clinical and operational processes.

APPLICATION

A single application will be submitted for the system.

WRITTEN DOCUMENTATION

Each component entity, a stand-alone group that is part of a multihospital or diversified single hospital system, must submit written documentation addressing each required source of evidence with examples occurring within that entity. For the purposes of the Magnet Recognition Program, the number of component entities within a system is equal to the number of designated RN executive leaders who are responsible for separate stand-alone groups within that system. This evidence must stand alone to demonstrate the full implementation of the Scope and Standards for Nurse Administrators (American Nurses Association, 2004) and the existence of a Magnet environment for nurses in the workplace. The documents and exhibits compiled to demonstrate compliance with the system eligibility requirements must be included in the written documentation submitted by each component entity. A separate DIF must be completed for each component entity.

MAGNET DICTIONARY

entity

A stand-alone group, whether or not within a system, whose nursing is governed by a CNO or a designated RN executive leader as identified in this glossary and whether or not separately legally established as a for-profit or non-profit, corporation, association, sole proprietorship, or partnership.

hospital system

The American Hospital Association (2007) defines *system* as "either a multihospital or a diversified single hospital system. A *multihospital system* is two or more hospitals owned, leased, sponsored, or contract managed by a central organization. *Single, freestanding* hospitals may be categorized as a system by bringing into membership three or more, and at least 25%, of their owned or leased non-hospital preacute or postacute healthcare organizations. System affiliation does not preclude network participation" (emphasis added).

SITE VISIT

Each component entity whose written documentation is scored within the range of excellence will receive a site visit by the team of appraisers who reviewed those written documents. The Magnet requirements must be fully evident across each component entity and at every level of each component entity.

SYSTEM RECOGNITION

If a healthcare organization with multiple entities opts to apply for Magnet recognition as a system and if any component entity fails to meet Magnet requirements, the system will not be designated as Magnet.

BIENNIAL MONITORING

Each component entity must complete interim monitoring requirements with evidence specific to that entity. If during the period of recognition any component entity ceases to meet Magnet requirements as determined as a result of investigation by the Commission on Magnet Recognition (COM), the system loses Magnet recognition.

Formatting, Assembly, and Submission of Written Documentation

All documents will be returned to the applicant, at the applicant's expense, if not bound as indicated below and/or the pages become separated during shipment.

FORMATTING AND ASSEMBLY OF WRITTEN DOCUMENTATION

- Use a common, easy-to-read, 12-point font, such as Times New Roman, Arial, Garamond, or Courier.
- Submit single-spaced, single-sided pages, except preprinted documents such as brochures or clinical pathways.
- Number each volume beginning with page 1, exclusive of brochures or clinical pathways, within a volume.
- Limit the documentation to 15 inches in depth, excluding the Organizational Overview (OO) documents, binding, page dividers, and tabs.
- OO documents may be submitted on CD-ROM or hard copy.
    - If submitted on CD-ROM, items should be organized by individual files, numbered to match each OO item (e.g., OO1, OO2, OO3).
    - If submitted as hard copy, place OO documents in a separate volume, with each OO item identified with a tab.
- Label all charts and diagrams with a descriptive title.
- Make all photocopies readable.
- Identify sections with tabs that are clearly marked and visible when the volumes are closed.
- Include a comprehensive table of contents with page numbers.
- Submit examples or exhibits in support of the narrative statement. If examples or exhibits are used once, they must be included in the same volume as the narrative. If an exhibit is referred to multiple times, it should appear in a separate cross-referenced volume.
- Paginate the cross-referenced volumes sequentially.
- Define acronyms and abbreviations upon first use in the written documentation, and include them in a detached glossary.
- Print the glossary on a color of paper that is easily read and easily distinguished.
- Insert the stapled glossary inside the front cover of the first volume of the written documentation.

- Fasten the written documentation in volumes by a method such as comb or coil binding to ensure that pages can easily be turned as in a paperback or sturdy spiral.
- Volumes also may be submitted as cloth- or paper-bound documents.
- Loose-leaf binders, three-ring binders, rubber bands, metal rings, and paper clips are not acceptable.

PAYMENT OF APPRAISAL FEE

MAGNET DICTIONARY

ambulatory clinic
A facility in which people typically other than inpatients visit providers for treatment and/or health counseling.

- Your organization's chief nursing officer (CNO) will receive an invoice for the appraisal fee (based on licensed bed size and presence of hospice, home care, and ambulatory clinics, if applicable) prior to your written documentation submission date.
- Mail the appraisal fee, payable to ANCC (*not* ANA), to:
  American Nurses Credentialing Center, PO Box 79120, Baltimore, MD 21279-0120.
- If the appraisal fee check is sent via FedEx, the address is:
  SunTrust, Attention: Lock Box Services #79120, 1000 Stewart Avenue, Glen Burnie, MD 21061-3209.
- **DO NOT SEND written documentation to the addresses above.**

PAYMENT OF WRITTEN DOCUMENTATION FEE

- A second invoice will be sent to your organization's CNO when you receive confirmation of your appraisal team.
- Mail the written documentation fee, payable to ANCC (*not* ANA), to:
  American Nurses Credentialing Center, PO Box 79120, Baltimore, MD 21279-0120.
- If the written documentation fee check is sent via FedEx, the address is:
  SunTrust, Attention: Lock Box Services #79120, 1000 Stewart Avenue, Glen Burnie, MD 21061-3209.
- **DO NOT SEND written documentation to the addresses above.**

SUBMISSION OF WRITTEN DOCUMENTATION

- The Magnet Program Office will provide your organization with the name and address of each appraiser selected to review your documents.
- Send one copy of the written documents to the Magnet Program Office:
  ANCC, Magnet Recognition Program, 8515 Georgia Avenue, Suite 400, Silver Spring, MD 20910.
- Additional copies should be sent to each appraiser at the addresses that will be provided to you.
- The documents must not include any items that could be perceived as gifts or inducements to the appraisers. This guideline includes the boxes in which the documents are shipped.

International Application Guidelines

Global mandates to strengthen nursing, improve the quality of patient care, decrease shortages and imbalances in the nursing workforce, and improve nurses' professional development and health environment have led to increased interest in the Magnet Recognition Program. Healthcare organizations around the world are using the Magnet program framework to achieve excellence in practice, create healthy work environments, attract and retain nurses, and improve patient outcomes. The evidence required for Magnet recognition in the international community is the same as for the United States or its territories. The Magnet Program Office remains aware of cultural, regulatory, environmental, and social factors in other nations that affect the practice of nursing.

CULTURAL TRANSFERABILITY OF THE SOURCES OF EVIDENCE

The Magnet Program Office conducts an in-depth conference call with the organization as a step in the application process to validate eligibility to apply for recognition. Using a dedicated international team of analysts and specialists, conference calls are periodically scheduled to assure organizations understand and accurately interpret the intent of the Sources of Evidence. A cadre of international advisors assist in all phases of the application process to ensure country-specific consideration for cultural sensitivity, relevance, and applicability.

DATA COLLECTION REQUIREMENTS

The organization must collect data reflecting nurse and patient satisfaction and other nursing sensitive clinical outcomes at the unit level. Data collection requirements have to be compared against national benchmarks. In some nations this is difficult to achieve as there are no comparative benchmarks. The Magnet Program Office will work with you to determine the best source of comparative data.

INTERPRETERS AND TRANSLATORS

It is important that staff have an opportunity to speak in their own language. While highly qualified international appraisers are assigned for document and site visit review, they may not be fluent in the language(s) used by the organization. Mutually agreed upon interpreters and translators may be used during the site visit. The translators and interpreters must work for the American Nurses Credentialing Center (ANCC) through a services agreement as all Magnet materials and products are copyrighted and trademarked. The cost for these services must be paid for by the applicant.

CONSULTATION AND EDUCATIONAL SERVICES

The ANCC offers consultation services, workshops, and study tours to assist international organizations on the journey to Magnet recognition. ANCC consultants are talented, experienced professionals who use a customized, collegial approach to identify organizational needs and the strategies to best meet those needs in pursuing Magnet recognition. Services available include a gap analysis or readiness assessment and data collection tools to assist in gathering required evidence. Workshops customized to your organization to educate and enculturate staff or address specific gaps are available. Study tours, a creative learning strategy, provide the opportunity to ask questions, learn about best practices, and experience the Magnet culture in several Magnet-recognized organizations. Visit the ANCC web site at www.nursecredentialing.org for more information.